Mentoring Doctors

Mentoring Doctors

How to Design and Implement
a Junior Doctor Mentoring Program

Dianne Salvador
Dr Rachel Collings

Copyright © 2014 Dianne Salvador and Dr Rachel Collings
All rights reserved. The contents of this book are protected by Copyright. Except as otherwise permitted under the *Copyright Act 1968* (Cwlth) no part of this publication may be reproduced by any process, electronic or otherwise, without first obtaining prior written permission. All enquiries should be addressed to the publishers.

ISBN 978 0 646 91535 7

Published by Dianne Salvador and Dr Rachel Collings
For ordering enquiries, please email mentoringdoctors@gmail.com

Cataloguing-in-publication data is available from the National Library of Australia.

Note: This book has been prepared and published for educational purposes only. It is not intended as a substitute for legal or other professional advice. While every precaution has been taken in preparation of this book, the publishers and authors assume no responsibility for any errors or omissions, factual or otherwise, or for any losses or damages that you may suffer as a result of the use of information contained in this book. Every medical facility is different and the information contained in this book may not be suitable for your situation. Before relying on the material contained in this book you should carefully evaluate the source, accuracy, currency, completeness and relevance of the information for your purpose. You should seek your own professional and or legal advice prior to implementing any of the information or processes contained in this book.

Neither the authors nor the publishers shall be held liable or responsible to any entity with respect to any loss or damages caused, or alleged to have been caused, directly or indirectly arising from the information contained in this book.

The statements or opinions expressed in this book reflect the views of the authors only and do not represent the official policy of the Doctors for Doctors mentoring program or State of Queensland Department of Health unless that is specifically stated.

Templates and sample communiques as specified are © State of Queensland (Queensland Health) and used and adapted by Dianne Salvador and Rachel Collings with permission. Such permission does not necessarily constitute an endorsement by Queensland Health of the publication or any service provider.

Cycle of Caring reproduced with permission (Skovholt 2005).

STOP reproduced with permission (Harris, 2007).

Questions from *The Art of Powerful Questions* reproduced with permission (Vogt, Brown & Isaacs, 2003).

Graphs from *National Mental Health Survey of Doctors and Medical Students, October 2013* reproduced with permission (*beyondblue* 2013).

Cover design: Vetta Productions
Inside layout: Zephyrmedia
Indexing: Alpha Indexing
Cover models: Dr Hobia Gole and Dr Brittany Wong

10 9 8 7 6 5 4 3 2 1

Searching for Certainty
Foreword by Thomas M. Skovholt

> "...in medicine... The steps are often uncertain. The knowledge to be mastered is both vast and incomplete. Yet we are expected to act with swiftness and consistency."
>
> Gawande (2007, p. 4)

Congratulations to psychologist Dianne Salvador and clinician Rachel Collings on a wonderful contribution to the important field of professional development with their book *Mentoring Doctors*. This book and its paradigm-shifting Doctors for Doctors mentoring program will, in my view, have a very positive long-term ripple effect, like a big stone thrown in a body of water, on the lives of physicians, their families and the people of Australia. The authors have put so much effort, dedication and time into developing this program and then writing about it for medical students, junior doctors, senior doctors, mentor doctors, and hospital administrators. Bravo!

Daniel Levinson and colleagues first documented the power of mentoring in their book *The seasons of a man's life* (1978, p. 334). They intensively studied the life course of four individuals including scientist John Barnes. They used the word mentor from Homer's *The Odyssey* and wrote:

> "[the mentor] serves as guide, teacher, and sponsor with skill, knowledge, virtue, accomplishment... the relationship enables the recipient to identify with a person who exemplifies many of the qualities he or she seeks."

You, the reader, may ask why *Mentoring Doctors* is so important and what is the paradigm shift? Both the Levinson book and the vast amount of research conducted since its publication have set the stage. In addition, I suggest this view. What a marathon the individual runs in order to get to the finish line that reads M.D.! So many hours of studying, so much competition, so much discouragement with sprinkles of joy. How can a person describe the extreme level of focus, excursion, intensity, and the length of it all? Does the following fit as a metaphor in describing the practitioner's journey?

Matt Napier's 2013 walk from Perth to Sydney in 147 days... a year after he cycled from Perth to Canberra. How about the term 'rage to master,' a term used to describe children and adolescents who have a manic-like intensity and laser-like focus as they run toward mastery?

For the doctor-to-be, mastery in science and math is central. The pursuit of perfection brings levels of mastery. Knowledge development and mastery in science and math at the university level involves using increasingly complex logical, linear, sequential thinking patterns. There are correct answers and incorrect answers, and mastering the correct answers involves study, memorizing, more study, thinking and more thinking. There are right answers! Like Matt Napier or others who have made the cross-Australia trek, finally the ocean, or the end of formal medical classes, is within view. And the person becomes a junior doctor.

Then the ambiguities of medical practice emerge! Anxiety for the perfectionist medical student who always got the answers right if he or she studied hard enough and long enough. The ambiguity – labelled the art of medicine – emerges and roars because there is now the human world of infinite variety (patient and family members and doctor and nurses and other staff members). They call it practice, as in medical practice, because it is imprecise. It can be so stressful for the junior doctor who is being evaluated on unclear, seemingly shifting criteria. No wonder that the authors of the newly released *National Mental Health Survey of Doctors and Medical Students* in Australia in 2013 found that:

> "...the transition from study to work appears to be a particularly stressful period with higher rates of distress and burnout in younger doctors compared to more experienced and older doctors." (*beyondblue*, 2013, p. 6)

In this world, the junior doctor may feel embarrassed, overwhelmed, confused, ashamed, demoralized and more. Yet, in the traditional medical training culture there is no room for the expression of vulnerable feelings. So, 'impression management' takes over. The junior doctor wants to look good – competent, assured, in control, talented, brilliant... so that he or she can be admitted into the inner sanctum of the M.D. world. Unfortunately, trying to 'look good' does not, according to the expertise research, lead to maximum professional development. The novice must be open with senior teachers and mentors about one's areas of poor performance and use feedback to focus on deliberate practice. For example, this sequence of being open to feedback but not derailed by it is a feature of our research on master practitioners.

In a tradition of learning via criticism and hardening of the self, the junior doctor quickly learns not to open up… but rather to push harder and conquer more and try to look good. Feelings of professional vulnerability, or what some American students call the 'impostor syndrome', are saved for one's trusted peers.

In this void of traditional medical socialization, has now emerged a new paradigm for the professional development of young doctors in Australia… led by two women, Dianne Salvador and Rachel Collings. Throughout the world, women are making the professional world better for both women and men and those we care for as patients, clients, students, and advisees. The old male style is compete, compete, compete, and don't talk about feeling hurt, lost, confused, anxious, depressed, or embarrassed. Dianne Salvador and Rachel Collings with their Doctors for Doctors mentoring program are altering the conversation by boldly stating: Yikes! Support, understanding, and help can often be better for professional development… and personal well-being too. This is a big deal. The authors of this book have named it – the high level of stress for M.D.'s.

Cheers to, and for, Salvador and Collings on the publication of *Mentoring Doctors*! This book is easy to read but insightful, full of theory yet practical, written for junior doctors and also senior medical administrators, and most of all for doctors who still remember the confusion of the early professional days and want to mentor junior doctors. This book is so timely given the high stress levels documented by the sample of 14,063 doctors and medical students in the *beyondblue* data. Like a stone causing a ripple in the water, so much good, in wave after wave, can result from *Mentoring Doctors.*

Thomas M. Skovholt, Ph.D., LP is Morse-Amoco Distinguished Professor and Licensed Psychologist at the University of Minnesota, USA. His books include:
Skovholt, T.M. & Trotter-Mathison, M. (2011). *The resilient practitioner: Burnout prevention and self care strategies for counselors, therapists, teachers and health professionals.* New York: Routledge.

Contents

Foreword	v
Preface	xi
Acknowledgements	xiii
Introduction	xv

Part One: Understanding Mentoring for Junior Doctors

1	The Junior Doctor Experience	3
2	The Case for Mentoring	17
3	The Mentoring Partnership	25
4	The Mentoring Program	33
5	Mentoring Program Development Fundamentals	39

Part Two: Program Design

6	The 4-Step Design Process	49

Part Three: Program Implementation

7	The Role of the Coordinator	59
8	Gaining Sponsorship	65
9	Recruiting Mentors	69
10	Attracting Mentees	73
11	Forming Partnerships	77
12	Training 'Ready for Anything' Mentors	83
13	Mentoring Service Delivery	93
14	Communicating with Mentors	99
15	Information Management	107
16	Maintaining the Program's Profile	113
17	Evaluating the Program	117

Part Four: The Townsville Hospital Experience

18	The Doctors for Doctors Mentoring Program	135
19	Interviews with Mentors of Junior Doctors	147

Epilogue	173
Appendix 1: Coordinator's Checklist	177
Appendix 2: Worksheets and Templates	179
Glossary	207
References	211
Index	215
About the Authors	223

List of Illustrations

Figure 1	Levels of very high psychological distress by gender in doctors, the Australian population and other Australian professionals aged 30 years and below.	8
Figure 2	Burnout in the domains of emotional exhaustion, cynicism and professional efficacy, by age group.	9
Figure 3	Integrating mentoring and other strategies.	40
Figure 4	The Mentoring Program Development Model, representing the design and implementation phases of mentoring program development.	42
Figure 5	The Mentoring Program Development Model aligned with the five-term junior doctor year.	44
Figure 6	The network of support programs and services available to junior doctors.	45
Figure 7	The Mentoring Program Development Model, with a focus on the design phase.	49
Figure 8	The Mentoring Program Development Model, with a focus on the ten dimensions of implementation.	64
Figure 9	A timeline for completing mentoring partnership formation within a five-day intern orientation program.	80
Figure 10	Making the abstract actionable in mentoring.	83
Figure 11	The necessity of evaluation planning prior to evaluation implementation.	118
Figure 12	Combining the process and outcome evaluations for a comprehensive program evaluation.	123
Figure 13	The process and outcome evaluation in context.	123
Figure 14	The Mentoring Program Development Model, with a focus on re-visioning.	131
Figure 15	The charter of the Doctors for Doctors mentoring program.	137
Table 1	Examples of transformational conversations: using questioning, listening and informing to facilitate development.	86
Table 2	Examples of process evaluation questions related to program inputs, activities and outputs.	124
Table 3	The Action Plan of the Doctors for Doctors mentoring program.	138
Table 4	The Implementation Plan of the Doctors for Doctors mentoring program.	139
Table 5	The map of mentor training content for the Doctors for Doctors mentoring program.	141

Preface

Rachel's story

My journey as a doctor began at James Cook University, an exciting new medical school in Townsville with a strong focus on patient-centered care. Understanding the power of communication and relationships was an integral component of the curriculum.

Following graduation, as I continued on to my years as a junior doctor, I began to recognise the unique challenges faced by junior doctors and my interest and passion for well-being grew.

I remember one of my first days as an intern. Patients and nurses buzzing around me, my pager beeping continuously and a pile of paper work stacked high in my arms that continued to grow. It certainly felt overwhelming.

Medicine is a demanding profession. Junior doctors face daily pressures related to professional workloads, internal struggles to further personal careers, and situations that place them outside of their comfort zones. Amidst the shift work and long hours is also a need to establish a work-life balance, and find time for friends, family and personal goals.

I recognised early in my career that every junior doctor faces times of difficulty. It is imperative to develop the courage to ask senior colleagues for help, whatever the circumstance may be. During overwhelming moments, it is these relationships that make a difference.

This notion developed into an idea for a program where junior doctors could establish relationships with senior colleagues, who would provide advice, assistance and friendly support. These doctors would be mentors, as they had navigated the same obstacles themselves and had gained knowledge and skills to pass on from their experiences.

I took the vision for a mentoring program to the Postgraduate Medical Education Unit of The Townsville Hospital. Dr Carl O'Kane, the Clinical Director of Training, shared my enthusiasm for this important junior doctor resource and put me in contact with Dianne Salvador, a new medical education officer.

As a psychologist, Dianne had experience in designing support for helping professionals within government organisations, and had the passion and drive to make it happen.

We envisioned a work environment and future for junior doctors where collaboration replaced competition. Together we designed a program, and with the support of The Townsville Hospital administration, the Doctors for Doctors mentoring program was born.

Since its beginnings, the service has grown into a resource utilised by significant numbers of The Townsville Hospital's junior doctors. It not only provides assistance and guidance to those in need, but is an easily accessible resource for career advice and friendly collegial support.

The program's design and implementation processes were presented at various forums and the interest in the program from hospitals across Australia grew. Organisations began enquiring about how they too could follow similar processes. This motivated Dianne and I to write a book which would serve as a guide for hospitals developing their own unique mentoring programs, tailored especially to the individual needs of junior doctors.

Interest in our program continues to grow as teaching hospitals throughout Australia and beyond realise the value of mentoring doctors. From humble beginnings, our vision for a future of well-supported junior doctors is becoming a reality.

Acknowledgements

Many individuals have participated in creating this book. We gratefully acknowledge their contributions and give special thanks to Thomas M. Skovholt PhD from the University of Minnesota for inspiring our approach to mentoring and giving energy and endorsement to our work; Allyson Agnew, Principal Medical Education Officer at The Townsville Hospital for providing support; and Associate Professor Kerrianne Watt PhD from James Cook University for contributing valuable outcome evaluation methodology content to Chapter 17 *Program Evaluation*. We also thank the mentors who have graciously shared their stories in Chapter 19 *Interviews with Mentors of Junior Doctors*, Drs Harris Eyre, Joel Wight, Chris Aubrey, Jamie-Lea Whyte, Ching-Siang Cheng, Sean Chan, Matthew Oates, Richard Gartrell, Rob Mitchell and Anthony Silva. To our families and friends, thank you for your encouragement.

Introduction

- Are you considering establishing a junior doctor mentoring program in your teaching hospital?
- Have you made the decision to implement a mentoring program but are unsure where to start?
- Do you want to apply a proven model created especially for enabling junior doctor mentoring?

This book is for medical education providers at teaching hospitals who want to design and implement a junior doctor mentoring program, to offer junior doctors more support as they transition from medical school to the workforce.

The junior doctor mentoring program

During junior doctors' transition from well-supported students to accountable professionals, vulnerabilities emerge in the setting of new responsibilities, schedules, personalities and location-specific challenges. Junior doctor mentoring programs are uniquely positioned to supplement existing learning programs and well-being initiatives, provide accessible and relevant support for individual needs, and de-stigmatise junior doctors' access to care. Due to the unique challenges of medical practice and the intense pressures placed on junior doctors, the scope of mentoring within a junior doctor mentoring program extends beyond the development of work-related competencies and career progression, to also encompass well-being. A junior doctor mentoring program enables conversations that guide, inspire and heal, through trusting relationships between junior doctors and their senior colleagues.

The Mentoring Program Development Model

This book is based on our knowledge of the junior doctor experience in Australia, and our journey developing a junior doctor mentoring program at The Townsville Hospital in North Queensland, called Doctors for Doctors. Our model for program design and implementation, The Mentoring Program Development Model, is transferrable to teaching hospitals across Australia. It may be equally transferrable to teaching hospitals overseas that value supporting junior doctor development and well-being. We leave it to you to decide the applicability of our model.

The purpose of this book is to assist you in applying the Mentoring Program Development Model to the needs of junior doctors at your teaching hospital. The model produces a mentoring program that:

- is tailored for your setting
- spans a 1-year, recurring and continuously improving cycle
- supports junior doctor development and well-being according to individual needs
- encompasses junior doctor professional development, career advancement and well-being
- is self-sustaining, by graduating mentees to mentors
- promotes a flexible approach to mentoring.

Through applying this model, Doctors for Doctors has achieved over 80% intern participation as mentees in the program. Mentees use the program actively for goal achievement and passively as a safety net. The program provides them with a year-long mentoring partnership, offering support that is tailored to their individual needs and is easily accessible. At the end of the year, many mentees apply to the program as mentors, stating that they benefited from mentoring and want to pass on the favour. Mentors report that through the program they learn a number of skills, for example communication skills, that can be applied outside of mentoring partnerships, in their interactions with patients and in their personal lives.

The structure of this book

This book is structured to make the topic of mentoring program development accessible to you. It will enable you to build your knowledge of the rationale for the junior doctor mentoring program and the processes of mentoring program design and implementation. By the end of the book, you will know what to do and why, when and how, to have a program that produces effective mentoring for a target group of junior doctors.

Part One prepares you to learn about mentoring program design and implementation. It presents the contemporary junior doctor experience, including challenges, impacts and rewards of practice, with anecdotes and findings of research conducted by beyondblue and the Australian Medical Association (AMA). The need for more support for junior doctors is highlighted. A case is made for mentoring as a way of increasing support for junior doctors, responding to their individual needs, and filling gaps in existing support services.

The concept of mentoring is deconstructed and the partnership and process aspects are brought into focus. The mentoring program is defined as a strategy, network, context and investment. Understanding mentoring and the mentoring program are the prerequisites for learning about and developing a junior doctor mentoring program.

Mentoring program development fundamentals are described, giving a broad overview of the necessary actions for the mentoring program development process to produce an effective mentoring program. The Mentoring Program Development Model is introduced.

Part Two focuses on how to design a program specific to the needs of junior doctors in your setting. It offers a 4-stage start-up design process using the key elements: vision, mission, and action and implementation plans. It also outlines a design review process for enabling the program to continuously improve and adapt to change.

Part Three covers how to implement a junior doctor mentoring program once the design is complete. It begins with an exploration of the role of the coordinator. The coordinator has a key role in preparing for and carrying out implementation, and is fundamental to the sustainability of the program. What the coordinator does, managing the mentoring program, is distinct from what the mentors do, delivering the mentoring services.

A set of ten guidelines for implementation are included. They can be applied in your setting in conjunction with your design, providing ideas for each dimension of action: gaining sponsorship, recruiting mentors, attracting mentees, forming partnerships, training 'ready for anything' mentors, delivering mentoring, communicating with mentors, information management, maintaining the program's profile, and evaluating the program. The mentoring service delivery dimension is the centerpiece of the program and all other dimensions of activity are in support of mentoring service delivery.

Part Four illustrates the complete process of mentoring program design and implementation with a case study of The Townsville Hospital's Doctors for Doctors. It includes program history, design, implementation, lessons learned, and mentors and their stories.

Throughout the book you will find many questions answered about mentoring, the mentoring program, and the mentoring program development process, for example:

- What is mentoring?
- What is a mentoring program?
- How can a mentoring program improve the experience of junior doctors?
- How do you build a mentoring program from a vision of what the junior doctor community wants to become?
- What financial, material and human resources are required for a mentoring program?
- How do you teach mentoring to new mentors?
- How do you support mentors to continue to be effective in their roles?
- What are the challenges of having a mentoring program in a teaching hospital?
- How are expectations managed within a mentoring program?
- What tasks are required to sustain a mentoring program?
- How can you keep participants engaged in the program?
- How do you know if your mentoring program is making a difference?

How to use this book

The information in this book is not just for reading, it is for actioning. You have the option of applying some or all of the ideas presented and incorporating your own ideas. We recommend that you read the text, follow the step-by-step design instructions and use the worksheets in Appendix 2, being the *Vision, Mission and Charter worksheet*, the *Charter template, the Action Plan template* and the *Implementation Plan template*. By the end of the design phase you will have a fully developed implementation plan, which you can use in conjunction with the implementation guidelines to implement a mentoring program in your setting. You will find a set of plans from Doctors for Doctors in Chapter 18, for your reference and or use.

In the collaborative spirit of mentoring, we encourage you to use the information and resources provided to design and implement your program in partnership with your colleagues.

And remember the map is not the territory. A book can never fully capture the richness of the mentoring program territory. We hope our map gives you confidence to find your way.

1 Part One:
Understanding Mentoring For Junior Doctors

1. The Junior Doctor Experience

An intimate day in the life of a junior doctor

It's another early start today as I push through the doors of the hospital ready for the tasks ahead of me as a junior doctor. I have worked a number of long shifts this week, which has left me feeling exhausted.

There isn't really a typical day for me, which is what I love about my job. Every shift is different, challenging and exciting. My role in the hospital is dependent on my rotation but is always based on patient-centred care and teamwork.

Currently I am a member of the general medical team and I need to arrive well before my senior colleagues to prepare for the day. My first task is to determine which patients are under our care, that the charts are available, and that all results have been reviewed. Once my colleagues arrive, I take part in the team meeting where significant patient events and overnight admissions are discussed. The morning ward round then begins, and I'm just hoping I will be able to answer the clinical questions from my consultant today. During ward rounds I am regularly asked challenging questions about physiology, best practice guidelines and current research topics. Although I often feel anxious answering questions in front of my colleagues, I know it will motivate me to continually improve my clinical knowledge.

As I carefully document the findings of the round in the patient charts I compile a to-do list that I need to attend to during the course of the day. The list grows longer with each patient review: investigations to order and follow up, allied health referrals, family meetings and pharmacy queries. I ensure I am vigilant in making note of each patient's management plan as these administrative tasks are my responsibility. Not only are they essential to patient care but if not completed diligently, will reflect poorly on my job performance.

Once the ward rounds are finished, I race into completing the paperwork for patients being discharged, ensuring scripts, certificates, discharge summaries and follow-up plans are completed. I feel pressured by time constraints, and the need to complete all paperwork prior to each patient's departure. It is my job to ensure the continuity of care continues efficiently following discharge, for the well-being of each patient.

After navigating the chaos of organising ward patients, I race to clinic. It seems my pager never stops as I get requests from nurses to review a deteriorating patient and respond to questions about management plans, as well as a call from the lab notifying abnormal results. I often feel the breadth and depth of knowledge needed as a doctor is overwhelming.

Sometimes, no matter how organised I am, there is just not enough time in the day to achieve everything. This is where I need to fine-tune my skills of delegation and prioritisation. As a junior doctor, it is often difficult telling your colleague that their request is low down on your priorities list. It is often even more difficult asking for help.

I then receive a phone call from my registrar asking why I haven't ordered the chest x-ray that was requested to be performed urgently. I had forgotten about it, in all the rush of the morning paperwork. I race off to the ward to rectify the problem and redeem myself.

Just like all my junior doctor colleagues, I want to be seen not just as a good doctor but as an outstanding one, a doctor who is organised and efficient, a doctor who contributes to sound patient care.

While on the ward, I am asked to see a patient who is angry about having to wait for their ultrasound scan. I delicately step into the room and am met with angry questions and frustration. I attempt to use the skills taught at university about dealing with angry patients, though nothing can quite prepare me for the real-life situation. I leave the room feeling irritated even though I have tried my best.

I finish my evening by reviewing my jobs list, ensuring nothing has been missed, and touching base with my senior registrar. My day is now complete and I can finally head home.

The junior doctor featured in this scenario was not one but many, a composite designed to give you a feel for the rewards, challenges and impacts of the junior doctor experience. In this chapter we begin with an exploration of these themes, drawing from anecdotes and four key references:

1. National mental health survey of doctors and medical students (beyondblue, 2013).
2. AMA survey report on junior doctor health and wellbeing (AMA, 2008).
3. AMA position statement, Health and wellbeing of doctors and medical students - 2011 (AMA, 2011).
4. 2012 AMA junior doctor training, education and supervision survey (AMA, 2013).

The role of the junior doctor

The service delivery role of the junior doctor is predominantly administrative, serving as the crucial link between their team, nursing staff, allied health services and the patient and their family. An efficient and hardworking junior doctor is an integral contributor to high-quality patient care and a cohesive team.

A typical day begins with an early start, arriving well before senior team members to prepare for the day ahead. This preparation begins by determining patients under the team's care, organising patients' charts and histories ready for the morning ward round, and ensuring all recent results have been reviewed.

The next task is the morning ward round during which junior doctors are responsible for clear documentation in charts and compiling a list of jobs required for each patient. These jobs may include investigations, blood tests, allied health reviews, referrals and family meetings. These duties are the responsibility of the junior doctor to order, to ensure are performed, to follow up and to discuss with their senior colleagues. Ward rounds are often fast-paced and require high levels of organisation.

Throughout the day, attending to nursing and allied health concerns regarding patients takes place between rostered duties that are dependent on the rotation, but may include clinics, team meetings, consultations, admissions and assisting in surgery. Time management and duty prioritisation are integral skills required to cope with this workload and delegate appropriately.

Preparing patients for discharge is another important role of a junior doctor. It is integral to ensure all paperwork is complete, scripts are ready, discharge summaries are finalised, and important information is relayed to the patient and their general practitioner (GP). This aspect of patient care is essential to streamlining appropriate follow-up and ongoing management.

The exception to this typical day is the fast-paced world of emergency medicine. Junior doctors have an important role reviewing and treating patients under the guidance of senior staff. The potential for procedural skill and knowledge development in the emergency department is high.

The rewards of practice

Medical practice has many positive aspects.

The human connection

Medical practitioners play an important role in caring for the community. The opportunity to make a difference in people's lives is morally rewarding and satisfying. Practitioners not only have the ability to improve the health of individuals, but also to empower communities, promote public health and advocate for improvement in healthcare systems.

Job satisfaction

No two days as a doctor are the same. Medical practitioners have the opportunity to specialise in a variety of unique fields. The ability to tailor practice to suit areas of interest makes it an exciting and mentally stimulating profession.

Community trust and respect

In general, medical professionals are regarded highly within the community for their role in providing healthcare and support during times of need. This is a very humbling aspect of being a doctor.

Lifelong learning in a mentally stimulating profession

Medical practice is continually evolving. Working within the medical profession requires commitment to ongoing professional development to ensure that high quality medical care is provided to the community. This dedication provides a career of lifelong learning as well as personal growth and achievement.

Teamwork, colleague interaction and teaching

Medical practice involves a network of professionals. Working as a valued team member provides the opportunity to work alongside inspiring and interesting people, motivating personal and professional development.

The impacts of practice

The medical profession is a rewarding career, however there are a number of aspects of practice that are challenging and have the potential to impact on the general health and well-being of doctors.

Landmark studies conducted by the Australian Medical Association (AMA) and *beyondblue* have improved the understanding of the impacts of medical practice on junior doctors' health and well-being.

In 2008, the AMA undertook a survey involving 914 postgraduate year two (PGY2) and above doctors across Australia and New Zealand exploring the junior doctor experience. The results were astounding, finding 69% of junior doctors met criteria for burnout, 54% felt their workload was excessive, and 71% of respondents were concerned about their physical or mental health during the previous year.

AMA reported in their position statement, *Health and wellbeing of doctors and medical students – 2011* that doctors are at greater risk of mental illness, stress-related problems, and substance abuse than the general population. The suicide rate of doctors is also higher than the general population. Among doctors, depression and anxiety are common.

In 2013, 12,252 doctors and 1,811 medical students responded to the National Mental Health Survey of Doctors and Medical Students, conducted by *beyondblue*. The aims of the survey were to understand and raise awareness of issues associated with the mental health of Australian doctors and medical students, and to guide development and delivery of support services for the medical profession.

The survey revealed multiple issues associated with the mental health of doctors, including very high psychological distress, depression, anxiety, suicidal ideation, attempted suicide, work stressors, burnout, stigmatising attitudes and resilience. The analysis of findings included comparisons of doctors with the general Australian population and other Australian professionals, and comparisons of doctors by gender, age and subgroup.

The survey found that doctors suffer from greater levels of very high psychological distress, depression and suicidal ideation than the general Australian population and other Australian professionals.

Alarmingly, 24.8% of doctors reported having thoughts of suicide prior to the previous 12 months, which is almost twice the rate of the general Australian population at 13.3%. Approximately two percent of doctors had attempted suicide. This highlights a serious and largely unspoken problem.

In junior doctors aged 30 years and under, the level of very high psychological distress was significantly higher than in individuals of the same age bracket in the general Australian population as well other Australian professionals. Comparison of levels of very high distress within these groups, by gender, is shown in Figure 1.

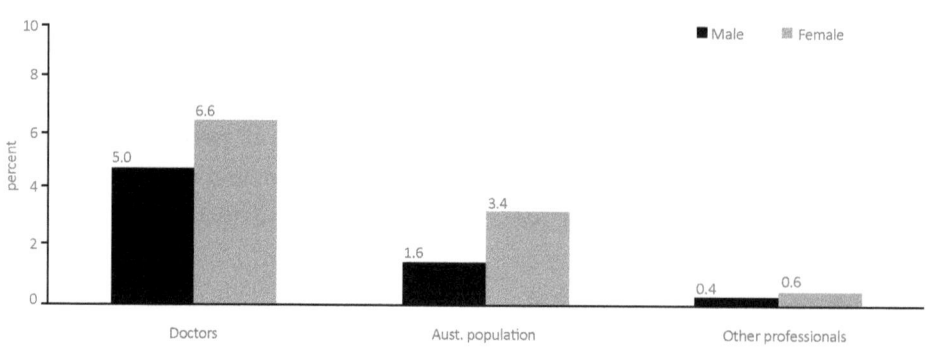

Figure 1. Levels of very high psychological distress by gender in doctors, the Australian population and other Australian professionals aged 30 years and below (*beyondblue*, 2013).

Compared with older doctors, young doctors aged 30 years and under had higher levels of burnout, with 47.5% of young doctors reporting emotional exhaustion, 45.8% reporting cynicism, and 17.6% reporting low professional efficacy, as shown in Figure 2.

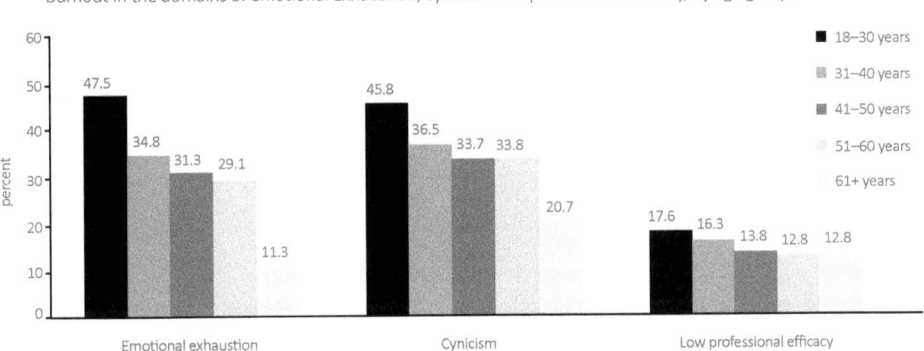

Figure 2. Burnout in the domains of emotional exhaustion, cynicism and professional efficacy, by age group (*beyondblue*, 2013).

Female doctors reported higher rates of general and specific mental health issues than their male colleagues. For example, 4.1% of female doctors reported current psychological distress compared to 2.8% of male doctors and 8.1% of female doctors had a current diagnosis of depression compared to 5% of their male colleagues. Similarly, anxiety in female doctors was higher, reported by 5.1% of female doctors compared to 2.9% of male doctors.

Indigenous doctors and those trained overseas were more likely to report stress due to bullying or racism than other doctor subgroups.

The challenges of practice

Work-life balance

In their 2013 survey, *beyondblue* reported that the most common source of work-related stress for doctors was the need to balance work and personal responsibilities.

Rachel says: Achieving work-life balance as a junior doctor can be difficult, and is predominantly due to a lack of control over free time. Roster challenges including last-minute changes, long shifts, overtime and shift work result in an often unpredictable schedule, making it difficult to dedicate time to activities outside of work. A loss of work-life balance has the potential to impact not only personally, but also on the ability to perform effectively on a professional level.

Home life

Commitment to the medical profession is often characterised by time apart from family and friends. Maintaining a life outside of the work environment can at times be challenging. Long and often unpredictable shifts have the potential to negatively impact on nourishing relationships as junior doctors feel divided between their personal and professional commitments. A stressful work environment also can impact physically and emotionally on junior doctors, which has the potential to affect personal relationships.

Relocation for training opportunities is common, and can result in professional, social and geographical isolation. The financial burden which follows many years of university can also create challenges.

Personalities

An often difficult aspect of hospital life is dealing with the variety of personalities within the hospital system, including both patients and colleagues. Some personalities are inspiring, while others can be intimidating and demoralising. Learning to deal with this array of individuals can be a challenge.

Career advancement and job security

Medical school and internship set clearly defined requirements essential for progression to graduation and subsequent general registration as a medical practitioner. Following internship and achievement of these requirements, junior doctors embark on their resident medical officer years, providing service delivery in a variety of hospital and community based specialties. These years are followed by application to a chosen specialty program. Opportunities and training positions are limited, and are distributed via competitive processes to the most elite performers.

Entry to specialty programs will continue to become more competitive as hospital systems become saturated with junior doctors, due to increased medical school graduates.

The 2012 AMA Junior Doctor Training, Education and Supervision Survey (AMA, 2013) identified that over the past decade, medical school enrolment has doubled. There has been an 80% rise in intern numbers from 2004 to 2012 and a two and a half times increase in vocational trainees in 2012 compared with 2000. This growth, combined with static supervisor numbers and unmatched clinical experience volumes, has the potential to impact on the quality of medical training and career development.

Professional development

A career in medicine is a commitment to lifelong learning. Engaging in ongoing professional development is a mandatory expectation and is another pressure faced by junior doctors.

Rachel says: Due to the rapidly advancing nature of medicine, a dedication to lifelong professional development is a fundamental component of being a doctor. Remaining current ensures the highest quality healthcare can be provided to the community. Self-directed learning accounts for the majority of professional development, and in most instances occurs in personal time. The most difficult aspect of ongoing professional learning is achieving a balance between long work hours, including a hectic professional schedule and time to commit to training and education.

Dedicated formal teaching for prevocational doctors is well-established in most hospitals, due to strict accreditation standards. Despite this the quantity and quality of the teaching provided is variable, and due to time constraints and administrative demands on junior doctors, attendance is often not possible. In the 2012 AMA Junior Doctor Training, Education and Supervision Survey, nearly half (49%) of respondents believed their hospital did not quarantine time exclusively for education and training on a regular basis. Interestingly, the survey also found that a large number of interns were 'not sure' of the structured education programs within their hospital.

Integration of informal or bedside teaching into everyday practice is inconsistent and dependent on the motivation of senior colleagues, staffing and time. With increasing demands on medical teams due to high patient loads and staffing constraints, delivery of care to patients takes priority over teaching.

Remaining current

Medicine is evolving rapidly, and it is essential for doctors to stay current with advances. Keeping pace with developments in medical technology, skills and knowledge, and changes in the administration and regulations of the health system, is challenging.

Assessment

Regular formal assessment is mandatory for junior doctors and is an opportunity to receive feedback and evaluation on performance, an essential component of professional development. A review by a supervising clinician is the most common evaluation tool.

Rachel says: Formal assessments are an opportunity for supervisors to provide constructive feedback to junior doctors and provide motivation for learning and improvement. Assessments should include highlighting areas of high performance as well as discussion of aspects of practice that require further development. Feedback should be sensitive and confidential to ensure the well-being and confidence of junior doctors is upheld.

Professional responsibilities and service delivery

The main role of a junior doctor is patient-centered service delivery and involves a number of internal and external pressures. These include being involved in complex clinical scenarios, the constant need to give to patients, compassion fatigue from the impact of distressed patients, and high clinical workloads due to insufficient staffing and hospital resources. This is often in the setting of feeling sleep-deprived and having limited time for extracurricular activities.

Caring for patients during their times of poor health, especially during end-of-life decision making, can be emotionally draining for medical practitioners. Junior doctors, unlike their more senior colleagues, do not have the years of experience in being able to cope with these common situations. This is a significant aspect of medical practice that can impact on the well-being of junior doctors.

There is also the daily pressure to be clinically up-to-date when dealing with colleagues and patients, and to be able to respond accurately in a variety of clinical scenarios, including stressful emergency situations. Doctors are often required to think quickly on their feet and the ability to recall important clinical knowledge is imperative to patient care.

Demanding workloads within hospitals have the potential to result in limited supervision and support. This can create additional challenges in relation to education, patient safety and service delivery.

Pace

Working in a hospital is fast-paced and busy. Although each specialty has its individual working environment, all junior doctor roles involve a significant workload. Junior doctors must develop the skills of prioritisation, time management and organisation to ensure daily duties are able to be achieved.

Team challenges

Working as a team member is a core component of medical practice. A team environment can provide support, motivation and a forum for sharing ideas. Challenges can arise, however, when a member is not contributing equally to the workload, or when there is a personality clash or a difference of opinion. This can lead to conflict and a stressful work environment, especially in a setting where colleagues work closely alongside each other.

Personality

Dealing daily with situations that have the potential to alter the future of individuals is stressful and demanding. Medicine requires a personality that is committed, competitive and driven to succeed in the profession. However, these attributes also have the potential to place high levels of internal pressures on junior doctors, and the aspiration to succeed can become overwhelming. The constant need to achieve contributes significantly to the high levels of psychological distress in junior doctors.

Transition

The transition from medical school to the workforce is a particularly stressful period for junior doctors. This is illustrated by the increased rates of burnout in junior doctors compared with their more experienced colleagues and also highlights the need for additional support during this time.

The challenges faced by junior doctors are vast and have the potential to impact on health and well-being in a continuous cycle.

Coping strategies

According to the AMA Survey Report on Junior Doctor Health and Wellbeing (AMA, 2008), spending time with friends and family is the most common coping strategy for junior doctors (29.2% and 30.3% respectively), followed by exercise (16.9%), taking time off work (6.7%), and discussing concerns with a mentor (5.9%).

The AMA's position statement, *Health and wellbeing of doctors and medical students – 2011* states that some junior doctors engage in a number of inappropriate strategies, including inadequate preventative care, not recognising signs or seeking help, self-diagnosis, self-treatment and self-prescribing, and delayed presentation to GPs.

beyondblue revealed that for doctors, barriers to seeking treatment and support for a mental health condition included a fear of lack of confidentiality or privacy (reported by 52.5% of respondents), embarrassment (37.4%), and impact on registration and right to practice (34.3%).

Who cares?

Very few professions match the intensity of demands placed on medical practitioners. The stakes are high. Patients' lives depend upon doctors functioning well, personally and professionally.

A number of organisations promote the need for protective and supportive initiatives designed specifically to address the unique needs of doctors. These are the cultural revolutionaries in medicine, who raise awareness of issues affecting doctors, identify gaps in support systems, and encourage the development of services specific to the needs of doctors. They include the Australian Medical Association, state-based postgraduate medical education councils, General Practice organisations, colleges, junior medical officers forums, and hospital-based doctors societies.

Despite the work of these groups gaps still remain in services for junior doctors, particularly in regards to support when and where it is required at work. Within your hospital you have an opportunity to address these deficiencies with a mentoring program catering for the unique needs of junior doctors. The program can provide:

- support for individual needs
- assistance with location-specific challenges
- someone to talk to when it is most needed
- feedback in response to "Am I doing well or not?"
- role modeling
- stress management strategies
- a focus on what is going well
- a celebration of progress and success.

Junior doctors need more support. This is especially relevant during their transition from medical school to the workforce. Mentoring can address gaps in existing services and overcome junior doctors' disconnect from support. In the next chapter, we explain how.

2. The Case for Mentoring

There are vast differences in the ways hospitals support and meet developmental needs of junior doctors across settings. There are also significant differences in the ways medical schools prepare students for medical practice and place emphasis on certain skills.

The AMA recommends that hospitals, governments and colleges support junior doctors by:

- ensuring access to confidential and high-quality medical and health services
- establishing professional debriefing, support and mentorship
- promoting access to early and expert assistance from professional services and providers
- establishing clear referral pathways for junior doctors in need of assistance
- adopting a 'no-blame' culture that supports those in difficulty, so that junior doctors are confident that seeking help will not damage their career progression (AMA, 2011).

beyondblue recommends additional support for younger doctors through specific mental health services, strengthened mentor-mentee relationships, and training to maintain well-being and stress management (*beyondblue*, 2013).

The mentoring solution

Mentoring can meet junior doctor development and well-being needs and satisfy each of the AMA and *beyondblue* recommendations in ways that other support services cannot. In this chapter we highlight and explain a range of benefits of mentoring for junior doctors that sets mentoring apart from other forms of support.

Breadth of support

Mentoring can address a breadth of issues for junior doctors including provision of debriefing, career advancement advice, psychological support, support for goal achievement, informal feedback and assistance with simple day-to-day concerns, all in one service.

Targeted support

Medical schools and internships based on the Australian Curriculum Framework for Junior Doctors (Confederation of Postgraduate Medical Education Councils, 2006) are generic education services. These pathways meet junior doctor population learning needs but cannot realistically cater for all individual learning needs. It is up to junior doctors to individually seek out extra commitments and learning endeavors dependent on their individual needs and interests.

Mentoring is not a generic education service. Rather, it is tailored to the needs of individuals with goals established by the mentees themselves. Mentors can give attention to individual learning needs and goals, including clinical skills and processes most commonly used by junior doctors, such as:

- time management
- organisation
- communication
- teamwork.

These clinical skills and processes form the foundation for achieving the predominantly administrative duties expected of a junior team member. As junior doctors progress, they develop knowledge, practical abilities, reasoning and clinical judgment, through hands-on experience.

Continuity

Junior doctors gain new supervisors frequently throughout the year. Short terms last only five weeks. A relationship with a mentor can span a full twelve months or more, enabling steady access to input and feedback from a senior colleague.

Understanding

In hospital-based mentoring, mentors work in the same environment as mentees, and most likely progressed through the hospital system as junior doctors. This provides them with added insight into the challenges and concerns the mentees are facing. With this also comes added insight into ways these concerns can be addressed. They have knowledge of the way that the hospital works, knowledge of the staff members, and knowledge of the logistical issues. These are all assets in the mentors' ability to assist mentees in resolving any concerns.

Constructive responses

Mentors participate in training that further equips them to respond constructively to junior doctors. Having a mentor means having someone available to give informal feedback; sometimes this may include a gentle reality check from a professional, objective vantage point.

Access

Hospital-based mentoring gives junior doctors ready access to support from mentors within the hospital setting. This is the winning component of the mentoring program that other services cannot provide. Hospital-based mentoring also allows the opportunity for impromptu catch-ups when mentor and mentee are both in the tea room, doctors' room, corridor, or other informal settings.

Education

Teaching hospitals provide dedicated formal training for junior doctors. Due to high workloads, time constraints and the administrative demands on junior doctors, attending formal teaching is often difficult. Furthermore, the quality of the teaching is variable. With respect to informal teaching from senior colleagues, this is dependent on the rotation and the registrar and consultant within the team. Mentoring can supplement this teaching.

Mentoring also supports junior doctor skill development in areas that often are not formally taught, like organisation, teamwork and logistical tasks. Mentors can play a role in assisting junior doctors to recognise where and how improvements can be made. Most junior doctors could benefit from guidance and assistance in at least one aspect of their professional skill set.

Two areas of need for improved education and training highlighted by the AMA Junior Doctor Training, Education and Supervision Survey (AMA, 2013) are in relation to teaching skills and research skills. Junior doctors need teaching skills to fulfill their professional obligation to educate less-experienced colleagues and medical students. They need research skills to review literature, design studies and assist with the translation of research findings into clinical practice. Mentors who have expertise in these areas are able to assist their mentees to develop as educators and researchers.

Off-the-radar feedback

Through mentoring, mentees can obtain feedback without the usual fear factor. Mentees appreciate the opportunity to check in with mentors and ask, "Am I doing okay?" and to have that conversation in a relationship separate from official assessment processes. The role of mentor is intended to be separate from the role of an education supervisor, who is responsible for providing formal feedback and assessment of junior doctor skills and performance. Formal feedback and assessment can have professional ramifications. Mentoring disconnects feedback from professional ramifications. The only exception is in relation to notifiable conduct, which, by law, must be reported.

Systemic changes

Mentoring cannot fix everything, but in cases where mentoring cannot help, mentors often can. We refer to problems within a system that can improve with advocacy by people who care, like mentors, such as the following examples:

1. Unplanned leave management practices.
   Many hospitals rely on junior doctors to mitigate the effects of doctors' unplanned leave on service provision. When colleagues take unplanned leave, junior doctors may be asked to provide extra cover for services by working more hours, giving up planned leave, and/or working at higher intensity. Junior doctors feel compelled to add to their workload to ensure a service remains operational.

2. Career advancement when there is no one to fill the junior doctor role.
   If a junior doctor is qualified and ready to progress to a vacant position at the next level of seniority but cannot be released from their existing job due to a lack of backfill, their career advancement stalls.

3. Assessment processes within hospitals.
   If assessment is done poorly or in an insensitive way, the impacts on doctors can be severe. Assessment is an opportunity to receive constructive feedback, to discuss areas of practice that are positive, and to review areas in need of improvement. It is an essential component of professional development. The assessor is integral to making assessment a positive experience, and hospitals play an important role in ensuring supervisors are carefully selected to provide appropriate feedback that is not only constructive but also sensitive.

We believe that the hospital should promote these assessments to junior doctors and supervisors as a positive aspect of career development, and deliver training for supervisors on how to provide assessments appropriately. Perhaps the mentor team could be involved in organising an assessor training night or helping to select senior doctors who are effective assessors.

Mentors can be agents for change in many ways.

Possible results of mentoring

Does it work?

To answer this question, let us return to the purpose of mentoring, junior doctor development and well-being, as our reference point.

Mentoring can and does improve development and well-being in doctors. For example, mentoring has been shown to help with stress reduction and adaptation to change (MacLeod, 2007). This could be the result of actively focusing on well-being and work-life balance during mentoring. Sometimes simply knowing that support is available can be reassuring and protective for a mentee, and can prevent stress or exacerbation of stress.

In a systematic review article published in the *Journal of the American Medical Association*, mentoring was recognised as a key component for career success and as a catalyst for career selection, advancement and productivity (Sambunjak, Straus & Marusic, 2006). A mentee who has made an effort to develop with the support of a mentor is likely to have broader networks and access to resources, strong skills, effective job performance and satisfaction, and positive working relationships with colleagues. Strong skills can result in good reviews required for training programs, job applications, and career advancement. Skilled, connected candidates get jobs.

Rachel says: "Careful consideration must be placed on appropriate matching of mentees to mentors. There are a are a number of advantages that can be gained through mentorship by a colleague within a mentees area of medical interest. This mentoring partnership not only has the potential to provide general advice to the junior doctor, but also the opportunity to provide insight into improving skills and qualities to gain entry into a specialty area of medicine. On the contrary if a mentee is paired to a senior doctor who is involved in assessment and reviews, the mentee may be less likely to discuss areas of concern or underperformance due to fear of the impact this may have on career progression. "

The AMA Junior Doctors' Health and Wellbeing Survey found that 5.9% of respondents identified discussing concerns with a mentor as their main coping strategy for work-related stress (AMA, 2008).

Why and how does it work?

Because the response to mentoring is dependent on many things, such as effort by the mentor and mentee, it is difficult to pin down a cause and effect relationship for the development that takes place. A determined mentor and mentee in partnership may try many methods until they find one that brings about the desired results.

Key contributors to the developmental results of mentoring are likely to be connection and relationship, which create a context for development. Doctors are self-motivated and can help themselves. They have to be that way to succeed in medical practice.

Sometimes some space, permission and a reminder is all they need to help themselves. Mentoring opens up that space, gives that permission, and reminds them that they matter, just like their patients. Mentoring prompts junior doctors to orient towards what is important, to take action, and to be encouraged and reassured that they are heading in a meaningful direction.

When, and for whom, does mentoring work?

All doctors have the potential to benefit from mentoring. No matter what point they are at in their careers, there will always be someone who can motivate, inspire and impart knowledge, whether it is by providing tips or simply providing a space for debriefing or discussing concerns.

The junior doctors most likely to benefit from mentoring are those who are:
- new to the hospital
- international medical graduates
- from non-English speaking backgrounds.

The junior doctors least likely to benefit from mentoring are those who are not open to guidance or change, and those who make infrequent or no contact with their mentor. This makes the self-referral aspect of a mentoring program significant.

Ultimately, mentoring can work if both parties pay attention to results, continuing to do what works and discontinuing what does not work.

Potential benefits to the organisation and society

Mentoring can also benefit the organisation and society. Benefits to the organisation include potential improvements and cost savings in relation to:
- quality of care
- patient safety
- productivity
- morale and job satisfaction
- attractiveness of the organisation as an employer
- workforce retention.

At a societal level, patients and communities benefit when high quality care is given by doctors who are functioning well. Doctors who look after themselves also look after their patients better. Research has consistently shown that doctors with healthy personal lifestyle habits are more likely to impart these behaviors to their patients (AMA, 2011).

A culture of care

Imagine a teaching hospital where the sharing of knowledge and expertise is the cultural norm and readily given, where collaboration rather than competition is the driving force of progress, where conversations are constructive and lead to learning, insight and effective action, where a culture of care permeates the work environment, and patients do well as a result. How good would that be? This is not just wishful thinking; it is a real possibility for the future through mentoring.

Soon, we will explain a process for enabling mentoring for junior doctors at your hospital. But before we do, let's take a closer look at what mentoring actually is.

3. The Mentoring Partnership

Imagine...

You worked hard preparing for this moment. You completed training. You ventured out short distances into the field. You got the certificate that said you were ready for the real thing. You're on the outback adventure of a lifetime.

After days of hiking, the reality of it sinks in. You are hungry, thirsty and tired. Your companions don't want to hear about your thirst, hunger, and tiredness; they are thirsty, hungry and tired too. You can't stop because that will make it harder for them. Like you, they are trying to find their way through.

You reach an expanse of rainforest. It's overgrown, and to get through you must squeeze your way through dense and tight areas, stretching across the small creeks that are in your way. You finally break out of the jungle into a clearing. The delight you feel turns to dismay when you see you've arrived at the edge of a cliff.

There is no obvious way forward. The sky is darkening and nightfall is not far off. You hear a dingo howl in the distance. Your feelings of frustration and exhaustion give way to fear. You're stuck.

You look up and see a person standing on a rock surveying the area from another vantage point. Somehow, in the middle of nowhere, they have a calmness about them. You can tell from their demeanor they are comfortable in their surroundings and know their way around. You call out to them and explain your situation. "I'm stuck. Can you help?"

The person nods. "I know this place well. I can help you find your way..."

Mentoring de-constructed

What is mentoring? Because mentoring can mean different things to different people, it is important to begin with an exploration of the concept of mentoring.

Think of a time when you faced a challenge or an opportunity and you felt inclined to explore it by conversing with someone you could trust, someone who had been there before. So you called upon that someone and had that conversation.

Let us assume they responded to you constructively, and by the end of the conversation, you had gained new insight or you were moved to take some action. The person who helped you served as your mentor, and what just took place was mentoring.

> Mentoring is an important and productive mechanism for sharing knowledge and expertise between experienced and novice professionals. Mentoring also has the capacity, through dialogic and human relationships, to engender passion and commitment to purpose and cause, and, in so doing, open new directions and opportunities for thought and practice (Australian Public Health Nutrition Academic Collaboration, 2005, p.4).

We can distil this definition of mentoring to its essentials. Mentoring is a partnership and a process.

Mentoring as a partnership

In mentoring, the partnership is a trusting alliance between a more experienced professional and a less experienced professional; a one-way developmental relationship geared toward the development of the less experienced professional.

Every partnership will be different because each mentor and mentee will bring to the partnership their own personality, inter-personal style, abilities and interests, agenda, and ways of giving and receiving help.

The key features of the partnership are:
- It is negotiable. It is up to the mentor and the mentee to figure out the nature of the partnership, the roles and the limits of the partnership.
- It is a commitment to help when required.

- It is a safe place where development can happen.
- It is a gift of sharing and goodwill that goes from one cohort of professionals to the next, if mentees later decide to become mentors themselves.

Many variations of the partnership can exist across a year and across partnerships, for example, in relation to the level of contact and the type of interaction within the partnership.

Mentoring as a process of development

The desired outcome of the mentoring process is a developing mentee, personally and professionally. It typically begins with identifying a mentee's starting point and developmental goals, and carrying out a sequence of actions and interactions towards goal achievement.

What does it mean to develop? It means to bring into being, or to become more in some way, that is to improve, grow or progress. Developmental goals of junior doctors could include:

- learning
- clinical reasoning abilities
- insight
- competency
- sense of direction
- work-life balance
- identifying and using strengths
- confidence
- preparedness
- self-awareness
- mindfulness
- resourcefulness
- flexibility
- helpful habits
- boundaries
- resilience.

Development in these areas can enhance professional development, career advancement and well-being, and enable the doctor to:

- place patients as the priority at work
- have confidence in their knowledge and skills
- have insight to know their boundaries and when to ask for help (and be willing to do so)
- embrace challenges and change
- continue to improve themselves through professional development
- remain passionate about their work
- have a positive attitude and mindset enabling high functioning
- achieve work-life balance by ensuring time for themselves to do the things that make them happy and the things that enrich their lives.

For doctors, development is an on-going aspiration. Doctors do not ever really reach a state of complete development or preparedness. The medical profession is constantly changing, and as a doctor progresses through their career, there is always more adaptation and development work to do.

Mentoring roles and responsibilities

Mentors and mentees negotiate roles and responsibilities, but in general, the division of these goes something like this.

The mentor:

- assists the mentee with setting developmental goals
- identifies opportunities for development
- reflects and provides feedback
- shares what they found important when starting their own career
- gives a constructive response to a question or issue
- facilitates (makes things easier)
- artfully uses conversation/communication
- assists the mentee in identifying values and strengths
- connects the mentee with people at different levels of the medical community
- shares their understanding of unwritten rules and expectations.

The mentee:

- identifies developmental goals
- discusses developmental challenges and opportunities
- seeks feedback
- plans ahead and does their 'homework', that is, thinks about issues before meeting with the mentor, works towards agreed tasks between meetings
- checks in with their mentor on a regular or as-needed basis to take stock of where they are at and plan for the way forward
- asks questions
- accepts constructive feedback
- ideally, reciprocates by sharing what they have learnt from mentoring by mentoring others.

Mentoring scenario

We will illustrate the partnership and process aspects of mentoring with a scenario featuring mentor Andy and mentee Lee.

Lee, an intern, joined her hospital's mentoring program at the start of the year during orientation week. She decided to sign up just in case something she might need help with came up during the year. She was assigned Andy as a mentor. Andy sent an email welcoming Lee to the hospital and offered to check in with Lee each term to see how each rotation was going. Lee accepted Andy's offer.

Lee has been in medicine for about seven weeks and has started to dread attending the morning team meeting where handover from the night doctors occurs. The consultant seems to direct a disproportionately high number of questions to Lee and they are pitched at a higher level of difficulty than Lee is ready for.

Around that time, Lee encounters Andy in the corridor and they stop for a quick catch-up chat.

Andy: How is medicine going for you?

Lee: The work is great, and there's so much variety. I've learned heaps.

Andy: Glad to hear. Sounds like this rotation is agreeing with you.

Lee: Hmm, yeah.

Andy: Is everything OK?

Lee: Yeah, it's OK. But sometimes it seems like I still don't know enough. There have been a few times when I have been asked a question in the morning handover meeting, and I haven't been able to give the correct answer. I'm feeling a bit exposed.

Andy: Those handover meetings can be a bit nerve-wracking when everyone is looking at you and waiting for the answer. Have you had some times of getting the answer right as well?

Lee: Yeah, there are even times when the consultant is asking the registrar the answer, and the registrar doesn't know but I do. At those times, I don't say the answer, I don't want the registrar feeling bad about it. I just want to make sure I'm not the one who looks dumb!

Andy: So it sounds like you'd like to go into those meetings feeling a bit more confident. Are you saying you'd like to be better prepared for those meetings?

Lee: I would like that, and I'd probably feel a bit more relaxed about handover meetings if I could.

Andy: So what sort of things have you tried doing to better prepare for handover meetings?

Lee: I come in early every day and look at charts. If there's anything I don't know, I get answers from Clinicians Knowledge Network. And every time I see a patient, I ask my consultant questions if there's something I don't know, and I spend a lot of time in the evening reading more.

Andy: Is that helping you feel prepared?

Lee: Yes, I think it does help.

Andy: Are there any other methods of preparation you've used before that you think could help here?

Lee: I could probably make a point of getting to intern teaching a bit more often. That way I'd feel like I am doing everything I can to be prepared.

Andy: You could do that. One thing that worked for me when I was an intern was to participate actively in handover meetings by volunteering answers to questions that were asked to the group. That way I would be showing everything I did know, not just what I didn't know. I actually started to enjoy the meetings and felt like I was reinforcing what I knew and had a more solid foundation to build on because of it.

Lee: Thanks, I'll give it a go.

Andy: Well, I hope it goes well for you for the rest of the term. Give me a call if you get stuck. Otherwise, let's talk some more next term.

In this scenario, Andy helped Lee to pause for a moment, consider her current situation and her wish to be more prepared for handover meetings, and identify her options going forward. Andy offered Lee a perspective that opened up a new possibility for Lee to use her strengths.

Junior doctor mentoring is about a junior doctor having a compatible relationship with a more experienced doctor, and benefiting from insights and actions catalysed by the more experienced doctor's words, presence and example.

When one partnership becomes many: the mentoring program

Once mentoring goes beyond one partnership consisting of two people, to a set of partnerships coordinated by an organisation, it is time to call the arrangements a mentoring program. In the next chapter, we will expand our focus and look at mentoring partnerships within a mentoring program.

4. The Mentoring Program

What is a mentoring program?

It's a strategy

A mentoring program is a strategy for delivering mentoring to a chosen target group. Both the mentoring delivered and the target group reached, are focal points of the strategy. As a strategy, a mentoring program seeks to enable:

- participation by the target group
- ease of access to mentoring
- the required amount of mentoring
- a level of consistency of mentoring within the program
- quality mentoring in accordance with mentoring standards
- mentoring that has relevance for the target group and caters for individual needs.

Delivering mentoring to a chosen target group will typically require other enabling strategies to be deployed in support of the mentoring, such as strategies for recruiting enough mentors, forming suitable partnerships and training effective mentors.

It's a network

A mentoring program is a network of people working in cooperation with each other in supporting the mentoring partnerships to succeed. The mentor and mentee partnerships are the core units: the mentors offer artful conversation and role modelling, and the mentees engage, participate and develop. Other contributors are the:

- Sponsor, who approves funding and endorses the program
- Coordinator, who oversees the program, working on and in it
- Mentors' mentor, who is available to provide guidance to mentors as required

Representatives of other agencies, who share an interest in the program, may also provide additional support.

The network of relationships is dynamic, changing as people move in and out of the program, as the external environment changes, and as program priorities change.

It's a context

A school is a context for sustaining developmental and pastoral care relationships between senior and junior members of the school community for a defined period. The school context gives the relationships a place and a space to flourish. The physical environment and the resources (the place) are conducive to progress. The time that is set aside for learning and the atmosphere that is created at the school (the space) encourages participation. Without this sustaining context, developmental and pastoral relationships would be limited.

Like a school, a mentoring program is a context that sustains developmental and pastoral care relationships for a defined period. A mentoring program opens up places and spaces for mentoring, and creates a helpful climate of shared purpose, expectations and safety.

It's an investment

A mentoring program is an investment in the sense that it requires resources such as money, time and goodwill, with the expectation of valuable returns. Typical costs of a mentoring program to an organisation relate to:

- Staffing – Mentor, mentee and coordinator time.
- Training and networking events – Venue and catering.
- Incidentals – Stationery and mentor badges.

The numerous potential benefits to individuals, described in Chapters 2 and 3, become magnified at the program level and can have a compounding effect, potentially shifting culture within an organisation towards co-operation and connectedness. Because mentoring offers a preventative approach to problems, it potentially offers cost savings as a by-product. Potential cost savings could relate to absenteeism, productivity, use of the employee assistance program, and supervisor and administrator time.

A program evaluation can be used to ascertain the value of the mentoring program to stakeholders as an investment. We cover program evaluation in Chapter 17.

Why have a mentoring program?

You may already be convinced of the benefits of mentoring at your hospital. But what are the advantages of a formal mentoring program over informal mentoring partnerships?

For junior doctors, a mentoring program makes it okay to access support and makes it easier to access support.

Making it okay

Establishing a mentoring program validates junior doctors' needs for support during their transition from medical school to the workforce and also validates the mentoring program as a worthwhile strategy. This validation influences positive attitudes towards mentoring, so that mentoring is perceived as advantageous for becoming a resourceful, resilient, effective clinician.

The mentoring program becomes a statement that it is okay for junior doctors to talk about their experiences, to aspire to meaningful goal achievement, and to learn easier ways from those who have taken a similar path before. This message helps to de-stigmatise junior doctors' access to care.

As more doctors join the program, participation in mentoring becomes the norm.

Making it easier

In a mentoring program, willing mentors and mentees are identified, matched and introduced. Mentees do not have to take a chance on being rejected by someone who has no interest in helping them develop, or no skills in helping them progress.

A mentoring program has a number of other advantages over informal mentoring partnerships, including:

- mentors who are selected for their goodwill and good intentions towards mentees, and who are trained to respond constructively
- mentoring standards
- clear information about expectations and roles
- time-limited commitments.

How does a mentoring program work?

Coordinated support for the program

In a mentoring program the organisation plays an intervening role in facilitating mentoring partnerships; directly, through assistance with beginning, maintaining and concluding partnerships, and indirectly, through sponsorship, communication, promotion, information management, and evaluation. All activities take place within a coordinated system of people and processes.

A designated coordinator plays a key role here. We will explore the role of the coordinator in more detail in Chapters 5 and 7.

Agreements to cooperate

Multiple agreements are at work in a mentoring program; they are the glue for uniting disparate parts of a program into one unified, purposeful system. For example:

- The sponsor agrees to fund the program activities proposed by the prospective coordinator.
- The coordinator agrees to honour the commitments made to the sponsor, including recruiting and preparing participants, and evaluating the program.
- The mentors agree to abide by a code of conduct and align with the charter that guides their partnerships with mentees. Then they form individual agreements with each mentee to cater for individual needs.
- The mentees agree to participate in the program responsibly, as described in the charter.
- A mentors' mentor agrees to provide support to mentors.

A shared approach to mentoring partnerships

A unified mentoring program, with some consistency of mentoring across partnerships, relies on a common approach to mentoring. The approach we recommend is the Cycle of Caring (Skovholt, 2005). In his 2005 model, Thomas Skovholt proposes that there are three key stages through which an effective helping partnership will progress. The stages, applied to mentoring, are as follows.

1. Empathic Attachment
   Essence: an open-minded attitude by the mentor; a trusting, collaborative alliance with the right balance between professional under-attachment and over-attachment.

2. Active Involvement
   Essence: consistent, sustained caring for the mentee; sharing a vision of development and progress and working towards it through a balance of supporting and challenging.

3. Felt Separation
   Essence: A letting go of active emotional commitments; separating well and being energised in preparation for future mentoring partnerships.

The mentor can use this knowledge to consciously move the partnership through each stage, towards results for the mentee. The Cycle of Caring is applicable to each mentoring partnership, irrespective of the mentee's needs. In this way, it is an ideal approach for the mentors to share.

We will further discuss the Cycle of Caring in Chapters 12, 13 and 18.

Challenges

Implementing a mentoring program in a medical setting is challenging. What looks on the surface like a set of partnerships between two people, is complex when dozens of unique partnerships and many other stakeholders are involved, seeking cooperation in an intense work environment.

Challenges include:
1. adopting an unfamiliar helping paradigm: listening and asking questions to diagnose and problem-solve (medical) versus listening and asking questions to understand and facilitate (mentoring) (Doherty, 2004)
2. shifting from a competitive medical culture to a collaborative mentoring culture
3. making mentoring non-threatening in an evaluation-focused work setting
4. finding time for mentoring.

The solutions to these challenges cannot be one-size-fits-all because every hospital and every mentoring program is unique. Next we explore principles of mentoring program development and a proven model, which can assist in addressing many of these challenges.

5. Mentoring Program Development Fundamentals

So far we have looked at why mentoring is a valuable strategy for meeting developmental and well-being needs of junior doctors. We have also considered how a mentoring program can enhance and expand the value and benefits of mentoring throughout an organisation and shift culture toward cooperation and connectedness. For the rest of the book, we will look at how you can develop and implement a junior doctor mentoring program in your hospital.

We will start by looking at the fundamentals of mentoring program development:

- Understand your target group and their needs
- Gain organisational support
- Appoint a coordinator
- Have engaged, effective mentors
- Build the program from a vision
- Manage risks
- Treat the program as a year-long renewable project
- Position the program

These fundamentals are the necessary actions for the mentoring program development process to produce an effective junior doctor mentoring program. The mentoring program that crystallised these fundamentals is The Townsville Hospital's Doctors for Doctors, featured in Chapter 18.

Understand your target group and their needs

What is the current reality for junior doctors? What are their needs for support as they transition from medical school to the workforce? Recognising those support needs is a prerequisite for program development.

Needs of junior doctors at a population level can be identified by agencies and peak bodies supporting junior doctors, who conduct research to understand the junior doctor experience. In previous chapters we looked at some of the common challenges of being a junior doctor and needs that are not fully met by other support services.

Needs of junior doctors at a local level may differ. To understand the junior doctor experience locally at your hospital, ask your junior doctors about their experience and what they need and want in the way of support. If there is no obvious need, there is no need for a service.

Keep in mind that the needs of junior doctors are dynamic, not static. They are dynamic because the work and political environments are constantly changing, and so are the junior doctors. The needs of the junior doctors at the start of the year can be vastly different to their needs at the end of the year.

Gain organisational support

Organisational support is crucial because it enables mentoring to take place at times when it is needed, including in work time at the organisation's expense.

Your program must have relevance to the organisation to achieve this commitment of support. Your program is relevant to the organisation if it integrates with the organisation's other plans and strategies. In the example shown in Figure 3, a mentoring strategy is nested within a hospital's education strategy, and in turn, the health service strategy.

Health service strategy
Provide safe, effective and sustainable health services that patients trust.

Education strategy
Offer clinicians educational experiences to support evidence-based practice.

Mentoring strategy
Help junior doctors transition and achieve their professional development, career advancement and well-being goals.

Figure 3. Integrating mentoring and other strategies.

Integration with existing plans and strategies validates the mentoring program within the organisation. Without this integration, the relevance of the program can be called into question.

You can gain the support of the organisation through a successful business case or proposal. In Chapter 8, we explain how.

Appoint a coordinator

The coordinator works on the program providing direction and oversight, and works in the program carrying out and delegating all dimensions of action that produce mentoring.

Having a coordinator ensures clear lines of responsibility for the program and a single point of contact for enquiries.

If you have strong organisational and interpersonal skills and sufficient time to dedicate to the program, you could be the coordinator. For the rest of this book, we are going to presume that you are willing and able to take on the role of coordinator.

Your role will be explored in detail in Chapter 7.

Have engaged, effective mentors

Mentors are at the heart of the program. They deliver the mentoring services that are the program's reason for being. They are also the change agents of the program. Through changes in their mentees, mentors create ripples of change throughout the organisation. Without engaged, effective mentors, the program cannot proceed.

Mentors are most effective and engaged when they are suited to their role, prepared for their role, and supported in their role through appropriate recruitment, training and communication.

We will discuss these areas in more detail in Part Three.

Build the program from a vision

Building the program from a vision means starting with a *vision* (an image of a better future; the future you want to create for junior doctors), translating that vision to a *mission* (the work that will make the vision a reality), developing the mission into an *action plan*, expanding the action plan to an *implementation plan*, carrying out *implementation*, and identifying a *re-vision* (a suitable design for the next year of the program). The prerequisite for all of these is having a sound understanding of needs.

The sequence we have just described involves two distinct phases: design and implementation. Our Mentoring Program Development Model shown in Figure 4 represents these phases and guides program development. We will refer to this model throughout the book as we lead you through the design and implementation phases.

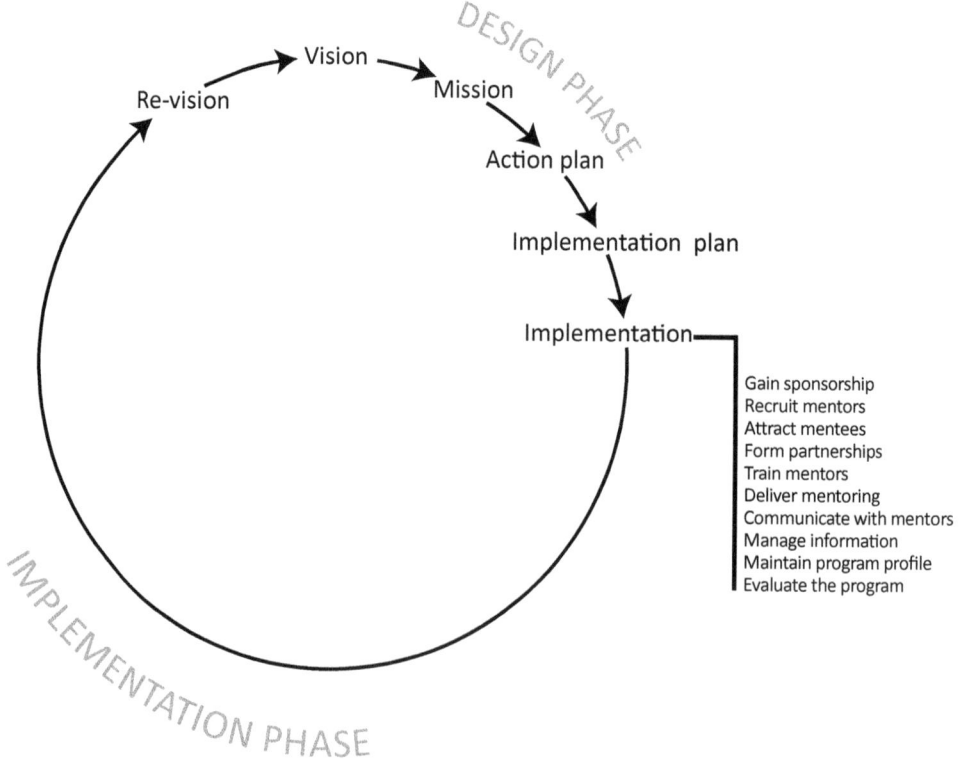

Figure 4. The Mentoring Program Development Model, representing the design and implementation phases of mentoring program development.

Manage risks

Risk is defined as "the effect of uncertainty on objectives" (ISO, 2009). In a hospital, uncertainty exists in many forms, for example work hours, clinical demands, funding and staffing. All of these forms of uncertainty have the potential to impact on the main objective of a mentoring program, the mentoring service delivery. Managing risk mitigates the effect of uncertainty on objectives. Without this, even the greatest mentoring program design will not deliver.

Managing risk will be covered further in Chapter 7.

Treat the program as a year-long renewable project

The junior doctor calendar apportions one year into five terms, usually spanning from January in one year to January in the next year. During this period, the junior doctors undertake rotations in various clinical settings with a changeover at the end of each term, which culminates in their graduation to the next level of seniority at the end of the junior doctor year.

A mentoring program which is an annual cycle sits well within this calendar. The significance of the duration is that a year-long commitment is usually manageable for mentors and mentees, and many doctors enter and leave the program and the hospital after a year. With the influx of new staff at the start of the year comes interest from people wanting to be involved in mentoring partnerships in one way or another, including newcomers who want to be mentees, and past mentees who want to be mentors. An annual cycle also allows you to review and revise the program each year for continuous improvement.

Figure 5 shows how the Mentoring Program Development Model aligns with the five-term junior doctor year.

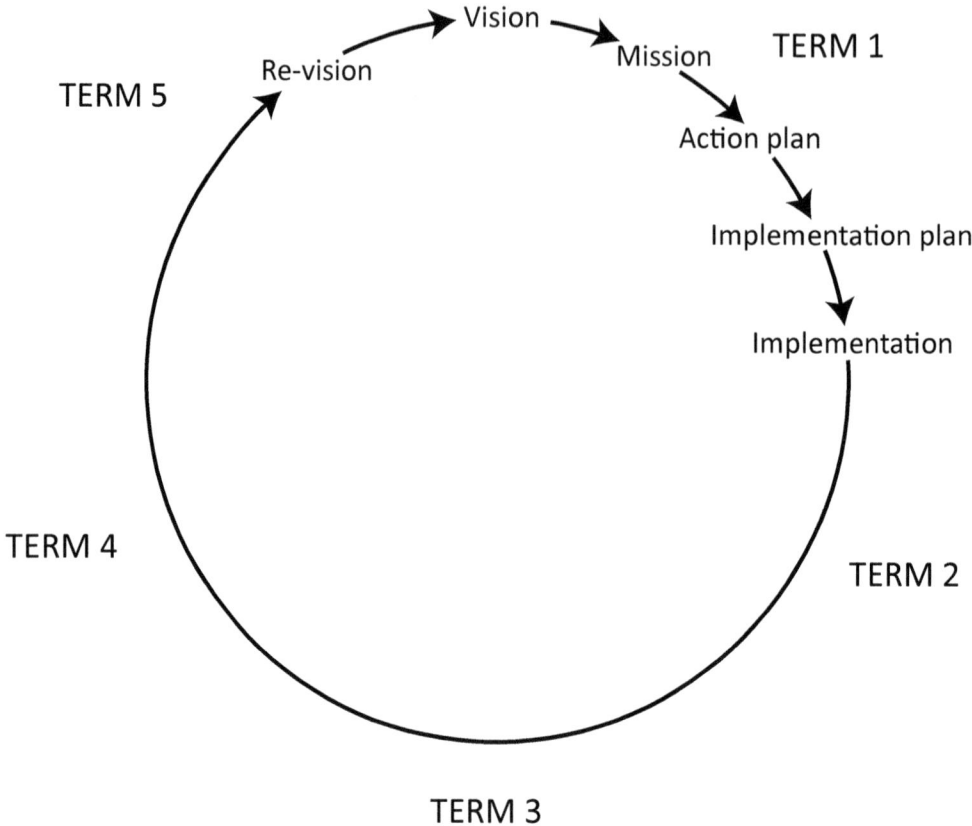

Figure 5. The Mentoring Program Development Model aligned with the five-term junior doctor year.

Position the program

An effective junior doctor mentoring program has its own niche within a network of support services for junior doctors. The mentoring program is intended to supplement other services, not duplicate them. In order to not duplicate existing support services, identify the boundaries of each service in your network and ensure that the mentoring program does not overlap too much. Figure 6 shows the network of support programs and services available to junior doctors.

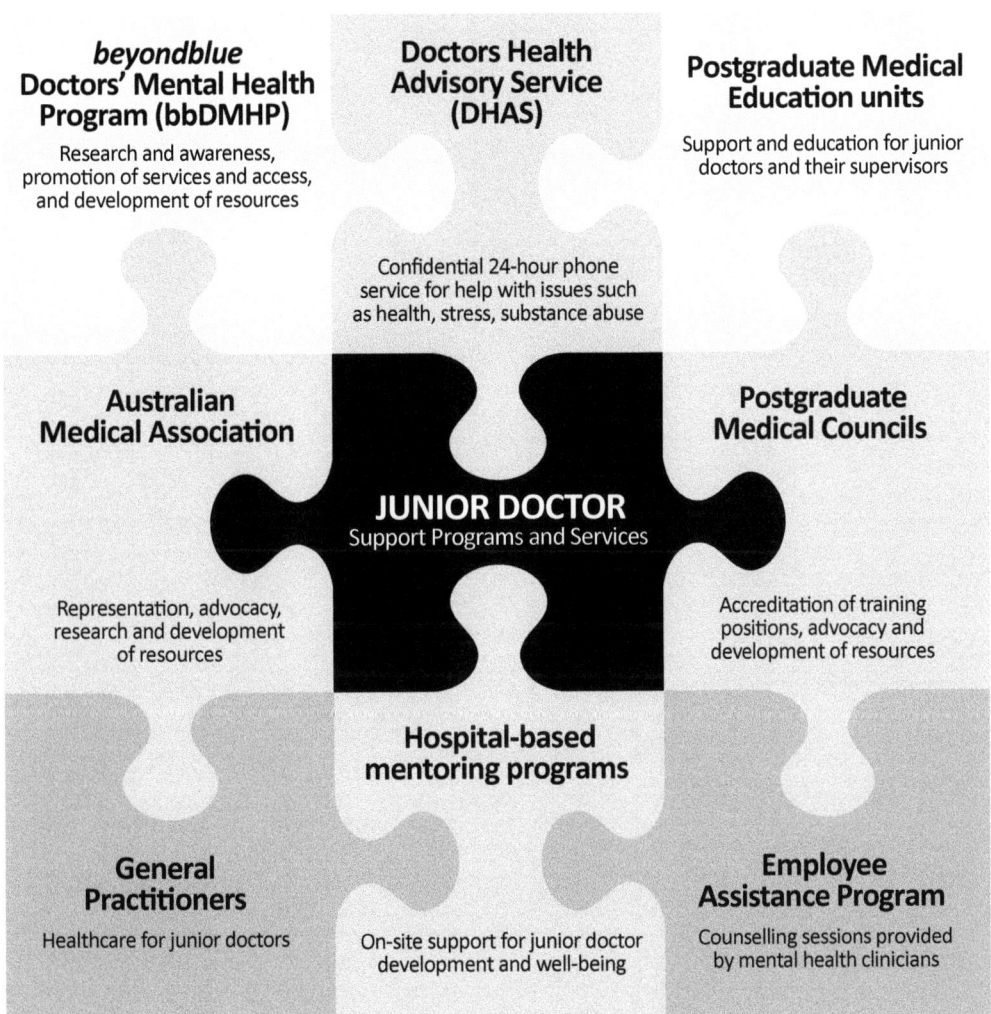

Figure 6. The network of support programs and services available to junior doctors.

Applying the fundamentals of mentoring program development

By applying these fundamentals, you can develop a mentoring program that offers relevant, accessible mentoring delivered by prepared and caring mentors. The program will have a defined place in the organisation and network of support programs and services for junior doctors, and will have the capacity to continually improve and adapt to change.

Part Two expands on the fundamental *Build your program from a vision*, with a focus on the design phase of mentoring program development.

2 Part Two:
Program Design

6. The 4-Step Design Process

The junior doctor mentoring program start-up design consists of four key elements: the vision, mission, action plan and implementation plan. The four-step design process is vision formulation, mission formulation, action planning and implementation planning. In this chapter, we describe the process of design, and we also explain re-visioning as a process of design review for programs beyond their first round of implementation. The design phase of the Mentoring Program Development Model is highlighted in Figure 7.

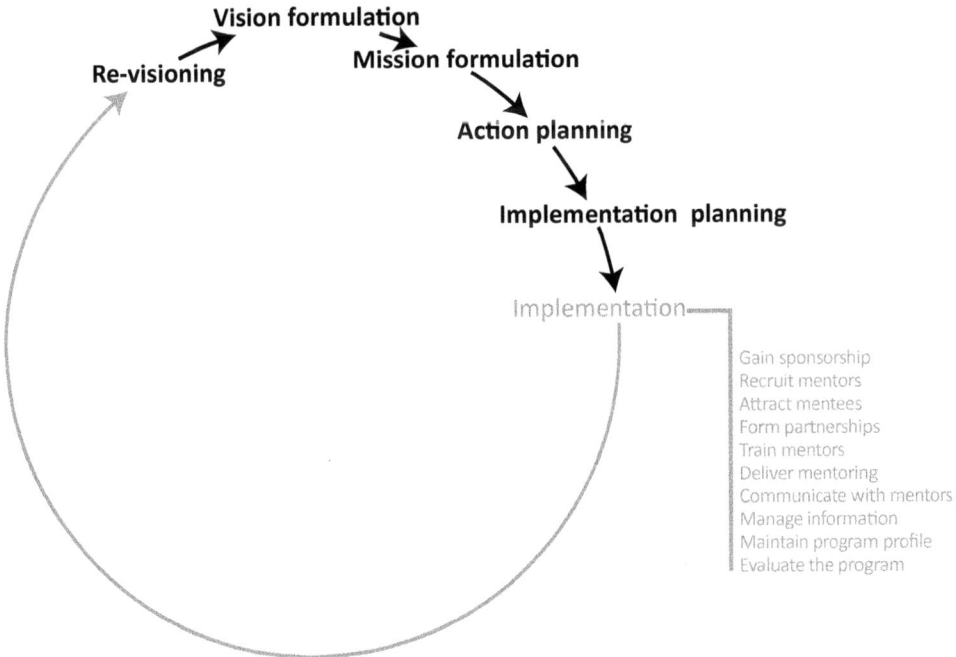

Figure 7. The Mentoring Program Development Model, with a focus on the design phase.

Step 1, Vision formulation: Start with a vision

A vision for a community is an image of what that community wants to become. An example of a vision for junior doctors is "Resourceful, resilient, effective clinicians." A vision serves many purposes. It gives a reason to take action. It prompts powerful questions about how to realise the vision. It generates inspiration and motivation, and, when shared, keeps everyone heading in the same direction. A clear vision opens up the possibility of realising a better future.

Some questions that can help you to formulate a vision for junior doctors are:
- What are your hopes for junior doctors?
- What future do you want to create for junior doctors?
- What does your junior doctor community want to become?

Ensure junior doctors are consulted during vision formulation, as this is a vision for their future.

Step 2, Mission formulation: Translate your vision to a mission

The gap between the junior doctors' current reality (their state of need) and the junior doctors' desired reality (the vision) is what you bridge with a mission. A mission is the work that will make the vision a reality. A mission is also like a program's fingerprint, identifying it and distinguishing it from other programs and services. For example, mentoring delivered through a hospital-based junior doctor mentoring program is the only service that can realistically respond with location-specific support to junior doctors when it is most needed.

A mission articulates the program's purpose and includes what the program does, how it does it, and who it does it for. Consider the example "We deliver to junior doctors timely and accessible mentoring for professional development, career advancement and well-being". This example articulates:
- what the program does, that is it delivers mentoring for professional development, career advancement and well-being
- how it does it, in a timely and accessible way
- who it does it for, the junior doctors.

This mission can make the vision of resourceful, resilient, effective junior doctors a reality. What mission could make your vision a reality?

There are a few more aspects and spin-offs to the mission that we will now tease out: scope, target group, values, and the charter.

Mission and scope

The 'what' dimension of your mission requires parameters. When we say mentoring is about meeting developmental and well-being needs, imagine how broad and all-encompassing that could be. Delineate your program's areas of focus, instead of trying to be everything to everyone. Set parameters, also known as scope, so that the service boundaries are defined and the target group knows what they can get help with. Scope also informs:

- selection of mentors who are suited to the role
- training of mentors to prepare them for the role
- the program's relationships with other providers of support services for junior doctors, who may be points of contact for referral or have collaborative roles.

Mission and target group

The 'who' dimension of your mission also needs parameters. Your target group includes only those who your program can serve best. Remember, duplicating services undermines your program by losing commitment from stakeholders. It also does a disservice to those junior doctors who need more help than your program can realistically offer.

Use eligibility criteria to define the populations and presentations most appropriate for your program, and exclusion criteria to highlight populations and presentations better served by another program or service. These will be explored further in Chapter 10.

Mission and values

The 'how' dimension of your mission reveals your program's values. Program values are the beliefs and guiding principles of the program, the ideals of conduct that you and the mentors agree to exemplify, and the essence of the program's identity. Values are timeless and are fundamental to your program. They speak to your target group about what your program stands for, and they serve as a reference point for decision-making within the program.

What will your program values be? Consider these examples and explanations.

Relationship – Connectedness helps.
Resourcefulness – Find a way.
Confidentiality – Protecting personal information.
Accessibility – Help is available.
Relevance – Making a difference, as determined by the mentee.
Flexibility – There's more than one way.
Creativity – When the answer doesn't seem obvious, get creative.
Strengths – We all have them. Use them.
Transparency – Be open about all aspects of the program.
Sustainability – Pass on the gift of wisdom-sharing.

Mission and charter

The most important program values are transferred to the charter, which is an extended version of the mission. The charter further develops how mentors will deliver their services and places emphasis on key values on which the program will not compromise.

This charter then becomes the program's commitments, so mentees are aware of their rights and what to expect from the program. We suggest that with rights come responsibilities, so it is reasonable to include what you and the mentors expect from the mentees.

The foremost commitment by mentors to their mentees is confidentiality. Emphasise confidentiality in the charter, and let mentees know from the start that there are exceptions to maintaining confidentiality, such as where notifiable conduct has been disclosed by the mentee, where there is potential for a mentee to harm either themselves or others, or where a court has ordered that the information be disclosed. Refer to the Australian Health Practitioner Regulation Agency (AHPRA) website (www.ahpra.gov.au) for more information about notifiable conduct.

Step 3, Action planning: Develop your mission into an action plan

Mentoring service delivery is the centerpiece of a mentoring program and the core of the program's mission. However, there is more to a mentoring program than mentoring service delivery. A range of other activities must take place for mentoring to be delivered to many mentees.

Let us return to our mission example "We deliver to junior doctors timely and accessible mentoring for professional development, career advancement and well-being". The processes required in support of the mentoring include gaining sponsorship, recruiting mentors, attracting mentees, forming partnerships, training mentors, communicating with mentors, information management, maintaining the program's profile, and evaluating the program.

An action plan identifies these broad dimensions of action and the specific activities that enable effective mentoring service delivery and sustainability of the program.

To create your action plan, list the dimensions of action and the corresponding activities required to fulfil your mission.

Step 4, Implementation planning: Expand your action plan to an implementation plan

After you have listed the dimensions of action and corresponding activities required to fulfil your mission, consider:

- Who will take action?
- What materials will they need?
- When will they take action?
- How will they know that they are doing the task or tasks to an acceptable standard?

By documenting your answers to each of these questions, you create an implementation plan.

You may decide to take on many of the dimensions of action as your responsibility. The exception is mentoring service delivery, which is the domain of the mentors. Note that some dimensions of action will be continuous, for example, communicating with mentors, and some will last for a discrete period, such as forming partnerships.

For most action areas, standards can be based on your choices of reasonable benchmarks. For mentoring, there are additional, specific standards you can use. These will be described in Chapter 13.

During implementation, let your plan guide you, but be prepared to adapt and improvise.

Re-visioning: Identify a suitable design for the next year of your program

After you have completed the four-step design process as well as implementation, it is time for re-visioning, the culminating step of program development.

Re-visioning is a design review process in preparation for the next year of the program. It involves checking the relevance of the program's vision and mission for the way forward, and making a decision to continue the program as is, to continue with adjustments, or to discontinue the program.

Re-visioning involves three enquiries:

1. Re-looking at the vision and asking, "Is this still the image of the future we wish to work towards?"
2. Reviewing the mission in light of the evaluation findings and asking, "Is this mission still the best way we know to make the vision a reality?"
3. Responding to evaluation findings by asking, "What, if anything, will we do differently next year?"

The desired outcome of re-visioning is a suitable design for the next year of the program.

You can undertake re-visioning as the final stage of the Mentoring Program Development Model after you have evaluated the program over the course of a year, and have identified ways to adjust the program for greater relevance and success. You can also undertake re-visioning throughout the year in response to changing junior doctor needs.

Re-visioning typically begins towards the end of one year as evaluation data flows in from mentees and outgoing mentors. This continues into the next year as incoming mentors join the program and make decisions about how they would like to shape the program and participate for the year to come. Re-visioning is completed when mentors share the same vision and mission for the way forward.

Each year new mentors will join the program. Many will be graduates of the program, that is, former mentees. They are a rich source of current knowledge about the junior doctor experience, and often bring with them original ideas for responding to junior doctor needs. Give them a say in re-visioning. In doing so, you will increase their commitment and improve the program.

You can think of re-visioning as a design shortcut for your program beyond the first year of implementation. The bulk of your design, that is, vision, mission and action and implementation plans will carry over to the next year of your program.

Your program

Use the planning worksheets we provide in Appendix 2 (the *Vision, Mission* and *Charter worksheets*, the *Action Plan template*, the *Implementation Plan template* and the *Charter template*), to complete your program design. Consider ways of incorporating the mentoring program development fundamentals into your program design. The Doctors for Doctors mentoring program design is featured in Chapter 18 for your reference and or use.

With your program design complete, you are ready for implementation.

Part Three focuses on the implementation phase of mentoring program development and begins with an explanation of the role of the coordinator in preparing for and carrying out implementation.

3 Part Three:
Program Implementation

7. The Role of the Coordinator

The role of the coordinator spans both the design and implementation phases of mentoring program development and is central to the sustained implementation of the program. In this chapter, we explore the role of the coordinator.

How to think about your role

Returning to the school analogy, the role of the coordinator corresponds with the role of the school principal. The school principal is recognised as the person who oversees the core business and support functions of the school. They ensure there are resources available to enrol and educate students, advocate for the school when required, and work hard on building and maintaining relationships within the school system and with related systems. Just like a principal, you will provide oversight for the mentoring program and implement all dimensions of action in cooperation with others.

Working on your program

As the coordinator, you are responsible for managing the mentoring program as a strategy for enabling access to mentoring, as a network of people that is oriented and moving together towards a better future for junior doctors, as a context for developmental relationships, and as an investment that is rewarding. To prepare for these tasks, you need the elements we introduced in Chapter 6. They are a shared vision, mission, action plan and implementation plan. Your work on the program begins with collaboratively formulating these elements during the design phase.

Working in your program

As the program coordinator, you are also responsible for program implementation, according to your implementation plan. This involves carrying out or delegating dimensions of action such as:

- gaining sponsorship
- recruiting mentors
- attracting mentees
- forming partnerships
- training mentors
- communicating with mentors
- information management
- maintaining the program's profile
- evaluating the program.

Note that mentoring is not on this list. Mentoring is the domain of the mentors.

The difference in scale between a mentoring partnership and a program is an important distinction to make. In Part Three, we will be exploring many different aspects of implementation, and you will need to be ready to shift your perspective between the partnership and program perspectives of mentoring. For the rest of this book, we ask that you keep in mind that what you do as a coordinator, managing the mentoring program, is distinct from what the mentors do, delivering the mentoring services.

Tools for working on and in your program

The three Cs

Your main tasks during the design and implementation phases relate to the three C's: communicating and connecting and then communicating some more. Let us look at each of these in more detail.

Every worthwhile program starts with the recognition of a need, a sense of potential, and an imagined better future for a community. Your communication work begins in the design phase by assisting junior doctors to articulate their needs, sense of potential, and image of a better future. Together, you have formulated a vision.

Your next communication task is to discuss and document the logistics of turning the vision into a reality through mentoring. You have formulated a mission and action and implementation plans.

At the beginning of the implementation phase your connecting work begins. First, connect the sponsor to cost-benefit information. If the sponsor pledges support, you can continue to connect: mentors to the program, mentors to mentees, and mentors to training resources. Once mentoring partnerships are formed, you can then switch your attention to connecting with mentors and ensuring they are equipped for their role. At this point, make a conscious decision to disconnect from the mentees and entrust them to the mentors. You have implemented your plans for gaining sponsorship, recruiting mentors, attracting mentees, forming partnerships, and training 'ready for anything' mentors.

The last 'C' (Communicating some more) includes exchanging information with mentors, showcasing the program to the community, asking and answering questions about your program, and presenting findings to your sponsor. Your most important communication task is recognising the goodwill and generosity of the mentors who are the essence of the program. You have implemented your plans for communicating with mentors, managing information, maintaining your program's profile, and evaluating your program.

Being the coordinator means being the architect of a network of people and information. Through communicating and connecting and communicating some more, you help make the program's vision a reality.

Forms

In this book, we will offer you forms, for example, worksheets and templates, to use in your program, with the disclaimer that forms do not make a program. See forms for what they are: tools, for communicating, for planning, for recording, for assessing, for collecting a volume of information quickly, and for remembering what you have to do next. Use these forms judiciously. The impression of solidness which they provide is just an illusion. The real solidness of the program comes from the strength and quality of relationships. Remember this point when deciding on where to place your focus.

Your priorities

Two overarching priorities in coordinating a mentoring program are supporting mentors and managing risk.

Supporting mentors

After the matching process is complete, you will have limited contact with mentees. Supporting mentors is the best way to ensure quality mentoring is delivered to your mentees. However, remember that there are limits to the support which you can give mentors. Scope applies here too. Enlist the help of a mentors' mentor to provide in-depth support to mentors in need.

Managing risk

In Chapter 5 we introduced the concept of risk. Risk is defined as "the effect of uncertainty on objectives" (ISO, 2009). The various forms of uncertainty in the hospital environment can potentially disrupt the achievement of the main objective of a mentoring program, the mentoring service delivery. Uncertainty can be in the form of:

- rostering
- work hours
- unplanned leave
- quality of relationships
- suitability of partnerships
- behavior of mentors and mentees
- preparedness of mentors
- potential resignation of mentors
- availability of mentors.

Uncertainty is an unavoidable part of hospital life. Anticipating and working around uncertainty improves the prospects of mentoring service delivery being implemented as planned. You can work around uncertainty using contingency planning. For example, you could prepare for the possibility that mentors will be occasionally unavailable at the times they have specified, by having an alternative support person available.

You can also seek to decrease uncertainty. For example, you could decrease uncertainty in relation to the preparedness of mentors, by offering mentor training.

In these ways, you manage risk.

An important aspect of managing risk in a mentoring program is a mechanism for resolution of concerns and complaints arising from participation in the program. Within the mentoring program, two supportive services operate: the mentoring that mentors deliver and the mentor support which you deliver. Things can go awry in both areas. What are your plans for resolving concerns and complaints? Consider preventative actions and responsive actions.

Preventative actions involve ensuring everyone has realistic expectations of the program and understands their rights and responsibilities. Your charter could include information about a feedback method. However, miscommunication and misunderstandings can and do still occur, even with the best and clearest information about rights and responsibilities, and responsive actions are called for.

With responsive actions, the aim is to resolve the complaint satisfactorily so that the two parties feel heard, understood and respected. Sometimes issues can be resolved with a conversation between two people. There are two sides to every story. Sometimes it helps to have a third person who can encourage that conversation and can be objective, looking at both sides of the story in order to suggest a way forward. Your hospital will have various people who could potentially be called upon to help, for example the mentors' mentor or the director of your work unit.

The ten dimensions of program implementation

Over the next ten chapters we provide guidelines for the implementation phase of your mentoring program, encompassing the ten dimensions of mentoring program implementation highlighted in Figure 8. Mentoring service delivery is the central dimension, being the mission of the program. The other nine dimensions support the mentoring service delivery. Our coverage of implementation begins in the next chapter, with gaining sponsorship for the mentoring program.

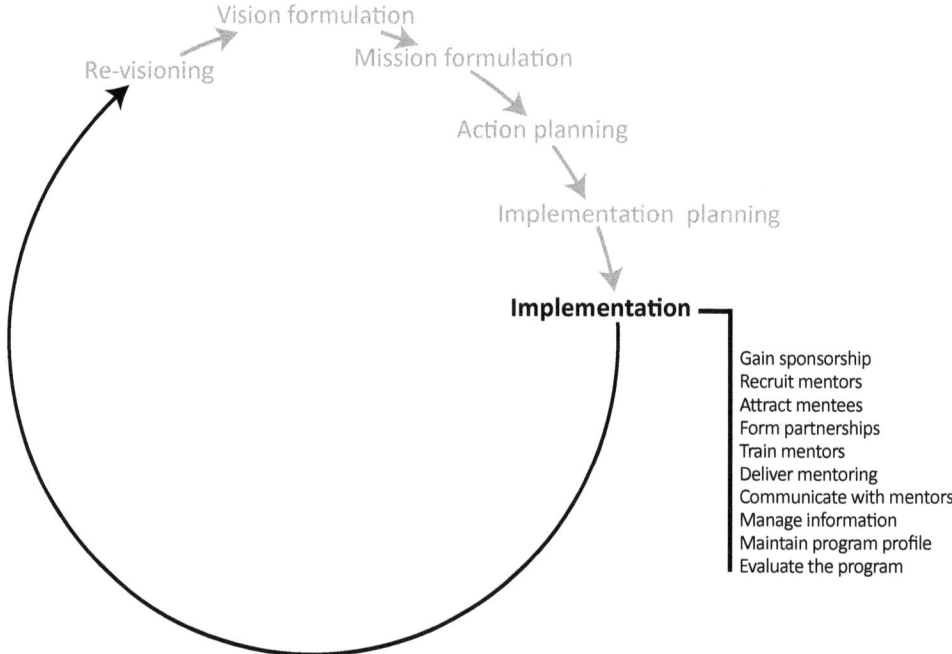

Figure 8. The Mentoring Program Development Model, with a focus on the ten dimensions of implementation.

8. Gaining Sponsorship

Implementation of a mentoring program begins with gaining the support of the organisation through a successful business case or proposal. Organisational support will allow you to run a legitimate program and assure participants that executive management approves of and encourages participation in the program. Without organisational support, the program cannot proceed as a formal program coordinated by the organisation and informal mentoring will have to do.

The sponsor

In this chapter, we will refer to a 'sponsor' and 'sponsorship'. We define a sponsor as someone in the organisation at a high level of seniority who has financial delegation, the authority to approve new programs, and the ability to give support on behalf of the organisation. In other words, a sponsor is someone who can say yes to the funding of your program and be a champion for your program. This is likely to be an Executive Director of Medical Services (EDMS) and or a Deputy Executive Director of Medical Services (DEDMS). If there are a number of management levels between you and the EDMS, seek their support of your program as well. When you take the case for the program to the EDMS, it helps if you have already gained unanimous support for the program and you have worked through any obvious objections to the program.

Know what you are asking for

As you take forward your idea of a mentoring program to people whose support counts, know what you are asking for. To have a mentoring program, you do not need much in the way of supplies. People and a place for mentoring are most important. Sometimes the best place can be a hallway and a wall to lean against. Apart from incidental expenses for stationery and promotional materials, and training expenses, the financial costs of a mentoring program mostly relate to staff time. Ask for approval of a defined amount of mentor and mentee time for participation in mentoring during their normal work time. If you intend to be the coordinator, ask for the role to be included in your substantive position, and for you to be approved as coordinator of the program.

Specify the duration of the sponsorship period. Although our Mentoring Program Development Model takes the form of an annual cycle, it is preferable to secure funding for a longer duration. This will allow the renewal of the cycle without interruption. A reasonable duration for sponsorship is three years at a time, with a commitment to report annually on the status of the program.

The business case/proposal

Making a case for your program involves giving the potential sponsor all the information they need to make a decision about whether to support the program or not. Essentially, they need you to present to them with the what, why, when, how and who of your program idea, and convince them that costs are worth it.

A sound proposal for a mentoring program contains organised information, the breadth of information that management needs to make their decision, and places sufficient emphasis on the likely returns of the investment. However, it is important to not overstate the benefits of mentoring when there are so many determinants of success.

For start-up

A comprehensive proposal is expected for a new program. Describe:
- what you are proposing (the strategy/potential solution)
- why you are proposing it (the need, the impacts of the need, the evidence for the solution and the alignment with other strategies)
- how and when you will take action
- who will take action
- the costs and benefits
- how you will measure its effects
- the risks and how you will manage them.

A proposal template is included in Appendix 2, *Proposal Template for Start-Up/First Year*. Note that your hospital may have a proposal format that you are expected to use.

After the first year

A less comprehensive proposal may suffice once the program is established if the executive management has not changed and is familiar with the program through your initial proposal and subsequent updates. Consider including in your submission these details about your program: what you are asking for, a description of the program's history and purpose, a summary of results so far, the costs and benefits, and a call to action, such as confirmation of continuation of funding. An example is included in Appendix 2, *Sample Proposal for Continuation of the Program*.

9. Recruiting Mentors

With sponsorship secured, you can proceed with recruiting mentors. Recruiting mentors involves identifying, selecting and engaging doctors who demonstrate goodwill towards their junior peers, the potential to be effective mentors through conversation and example, and fitness to represent your program.

Mentor motives

Doctors apply to be mentors for various reasons. Many feel inspired by experiences they have had with their own mentor. Most remember what it was like to be in the mentee's position, and think, "If only someone had told me (something they had to learn the hard way)." Some wish to gain experience in clinical teaching. Often their interest stems simply from goodwill for their junior peers. Sometimes it is a combination of all of these things.

Selection criteria

The only prerequisite for being a mentor in a junior doctor mentoring program is to be a doctor with an ability to have a developmental relationship with junior colleagues.

An effective mentor accepts mentees, works with mentees on their goals, uses listening and questioning effectively for many purposes including facilitation, and is fully present during conversations.

Recruit for availability, willingness, goodwill, good example (professionalism and work-life balance), more seniority than the mentee target group, and for agreement with your program's vision and charter. The rest, you can train for.

Keep in mind, diversity within a mentor group is advantageous because there is a similar amount of diversity in a mentee group. Diversity provides you with better chances of suitable matches.

Group size

Decide how many mentors you will need in your program to deliver your mission. How many new junior doctors will be arriving at your hospital? How many junior doctors are likely to want a mentor? What is your capacity to train and support mentors over a year? These are all considerations.

Attracting mentor applicants

To influence prospective mentors, communicate with them about the program, the reasons that you are asking for their help, and what you would expect of them as mentors.

Communication channels

You can use direct contact to reach prospective mentors. If you have ways of contacting doctors at a certain level of seniority, you can approach them as a group. Group email, as per the example below, is efficient for this purpose. Requesting an expression of interest from applicants will enable you to get to know the applicants and gauge their suitability.

[Name of Mentoring program]

Nominate now to become a mentor in [Year].

This program was established in [Year] to help junior doctors transition and achieve their professional development, career advancement and well-being goals.

Position overview:
- PGY2 or above
- Willingness to volunteer your time to assist junior doctors in need of support and guidance this year
- One mentor meeting per term

You will receive training and ongoing support to be an effective mentor.

To nominate:
Email your name and a short statement why you would make a good mentor to [Email address of coordinator].
[Number] mentors will be selected by the [Unit].

Deadline: [Date]

Get involved and make a difference!

© State of Queensland (Queensland Health) 2011-2013

You can also ask around the mentor group and the higher ranks of clinicians for their recommendations, and then approach those recommended individuals directly. Ideally, you will recruit from the mentee group towards the end of the year as they will have an experience of mentoring in general and of your hospital's mentoring program in particular; a good starting point for new mentors to build on. Consider giving the mentee group advanced notice of upcoming mentor recruitment, as per the email example below.

Dear Doctors,

Thanks for being part of the [Mentoring program] as mentees.

I am writing to encourage you to make contact with your mentor, if you haven't already. Your mentors are willing and able to listen, provide constructive feedback, refer you to resources available, and celebrate your successes. Later this year I will be inviting you to apply to the program to be a mentor to new junior doctors in [Year]. To become an effective mentor, it helps if you've been mentored yourself.

If you need to be reminded of who your mentor is, or their contact details, let me know and I'll send you details.

Kind regards,

[Coordinator]

© State of Queensland (Queensland Health) 2011-2013

Notifying mentor applicants of the outcome of their application

The process for selection should be merit-based. Advise the applicants in writing of the selection outcome, regardless of whether the applicants are successful or not in their application. If you are declining an application, explain the decision to the applicant and options for re-applying in the future. For the successful applicants, you can send an email such as the following notice of successful application.

---

* Congratulations, you have been selected as a [Year, Mentoring program] Mentor *

[Coordinator] will provide your training and ongoing support in [Year] and will be in touch with you soon with more information about the program.

Welcome to [Mentoring program] for [year].

Kind regards,

[Unit Director]

© State of Queensland (Queensland Health) 2011-2013

After recruitment

Between recruitment and mentoring delivery is a period of orientation for mentors. Following the notice of successful application, provide mentors with further introductory information about the program and what to expect throughout the year. This is also an opportune time to request information useful for matching and to form agreements with mentors.

Preparing for matching

To prepare for matching, you will need additional information about the mentor's background, availability and interest areas, for comparison with the mentees' specifications. A mentor biography form allows you to collect this information in preparation for matching. An example is included in Appendix 2, *Mentor Bio form*.

Forming agreements with mentors

A mentoring program relies on the trustworthiness of mentors in caring for mentees as promised and in caring for the program. Agreements confirm the mentors' commitment to care. Mentors are asked to sign off on their agreement to:

1. perform mentor duties
2. maintain confidentiality
3. uphold the charter.

Agreements for signing can be provided to mentors within an orientation pack. A sample *Summary of Duties and Confidentiality Agreement* is provided in Appendix 2.

The first meeting

At the first meeting, mentors have the opportunity to contribute to re-visioning, as per our definition in Chapters 5 and 6. This can be done in an informal, relaxed way, as shown in the *Sample First Meeting Plan* in Appendix 2.

10. Attracting Mentees

Once mentor recruitment is complete and the availability of mentors is confirmed, the mentoring program can be offered to prospective mentees. Attracting mentees is about gaining the attention of the target group, conveying the value of the mentoring services on offer, and encouraging registration in the program.

Know who they are

Junior doctors, or a subgroup of junior doctors, are the target group of a junior doctor mentoring program. The junior doctors will have a range of intentions for participation in the mentoring program. Some mentees may decide to get involved to have a safety net in case of difficulties, some may wish to be more actively involved in setting and achieving professional development, career advancement and or well-being goals, and some may be unsure about participating but are willing to give it a try. These are all reasonable starting points for joining a mentoring program that aims to be relevant to mentees.

Know who they are not

Exclusion criteria

Once you have defined the target group for your program, you may wish to form exclusion criteria to highlight those needs better served by another program or service. Exclusion criteria can relate to: a population for example, senior doctors; or a presentation, for example, substance abuse.

Referral

Referral is appropriate for mentee applicants who meet exclusion criteria. This will help them find the best possible alternative program or service for their needs, and also protect mentors from being asked to deliver specialised interventions beyond their expertise and beyond the scope of the program.

As coordinator, you can refer in response to a mentee application, or the mentors can refer during the mentoring partnership. Ensure mentors have a clear understanding of the limits to mentoring and have referral information to give to mentees who meet exclusion criteria.

Communicating with prospective mentees

Timing

Many prospective mentees are at their most vulnerable when they arrive at the hospital as interns. Some will have no prior experience of the hospital, while others will have spent time in the hospital as medical students. Whether or not the hospital is new to them, they realise that their level of responsibility is significantly changing, and they tend to be receptive to offers of help.

Interns' first week is orientation. Orientation is the ideal time to introduce interns to your mentoring program.

Channels

A personal presentation about your mentoring program allows you to directly provide information to interns about the program and how it can meet their needs. Your presence also allows them to ask questions on the spot, and gives them a chance to resolve any uncertainties they might have about being involved. Your challenge as a presenter is to be coherent and concise about mentoring, a somewhat nebulous topic. You could provide a useful metaphor by describing mentoring as a navigational aid that helps mentees find their way.

Essentially, mentees want to know what they will gain from being involved. You can explain that they gain a year-long commitment from a mentor who will provide support that is accessible and relevant to the mentee.

Mentee expressions of interest

A quick way of gathering expressions of interest from a group of prospective mentees is to use a mentee expression of interest (EOI) form. A sample is provided in Appendix 2, *Expression of Interest - Mentee*.

This form serves other purposes as well. It provides mentees with more information about the program and a means of specifying what they are seeking in and from a mentor. It also allows you to collect information about mentees in preparation for matching, including mentees' educational background and their intentions for participating in mentoring. With this information, you can consider the suitability of matches, as well as the number of mentees to assign each mentor. With this information, mentors can have an idea of the expected level of participation by their mentees, anticipate the overall demand for their mentoring, and make decisions about whether to approach mentees if they do not hear from them.

Involving mentors in a presentation, such as a Question and Answer panel, around the time you issue this form allows mentors to further introduce themselves and the program. Also, prospective mentees can identify and specify their preferred mentor.

Preparing mentees for productive mentoring

How can you prepare mentees to gain the most from a mentoring partnership?

To encourage participation in mentoring, give mentees ideas about the issues they can bring to mentoring, for example:

- challenges and opportunities
- the help they can ask for e.g. conversations and role modelling
- their rights and responsibilities as per the charter
- what they can expect (above all, confidentiality with limits explained clearly from the start).

While clearly-defined objectives or pre-set goals are an advantageous place to start, they are not prerequisites for a productive mentoring partnership. An attitude of openness and curiosity will do.

To encourage constructive conversations, equip mentees with skills for questioning, for example, building productive enquiries from who, what, when, where, why and how questions). Also, encourage assertion when responding to tricky or awkward mentoring situations, such as unwanted advice from a mentor.

11. Forming Partnerships

After mentors and mentees are accepted into the program, matching can occur to facilitate partnership formation. Matching is assigning one mentor and one mentee to a suitable partnership. It is done in a considered way to maximise the chances of the partnership taking off and supporting mentee development and well-being. Matching is usually based on qualities and interest areas identified by both the mentor and mentee in the application process. Your job is to compare mentee wants with mentor offerings and find the best fit.

For and against matching

The advantage of matching mentees to mentors, as opposed to leaving mentees to find their own mentor within the program, is that you have the ability to facilitate a connection between two people, when those two people may not have had the confidence or the opportunity to meet without that facilitation taking place.

One of the disadvantages of matching is that there may be things about the mentor or mentee that make the match unsuitable, such as personality differences or a dual relationship (a pre-existing relationship that precludes a helpful mentoring partnership), but you have no way of knowing of the incompatibility until the match is revealed.

Criteria for suitable matches

Mutual respect

The basis of a suitable match is mutual respect and a shared commitment to the mentee's development and well-being.

Meets specifications

If a mentee states they have no specifications for a mentor, they are saying that any partnership is a match. If they have specifications for a mentor, a suitable match would be one that takes into account their specifications.

Some commonality

During matching, you are looking for enough similarities to form a connection on which to build a relationship. Similar career aspirations and values are often a basis for a strong mentoring partnership. Finding one area of commonality is a good start. The commonality might be a university, interest, career path or ambition. Enough similarity can help the partnership get going; enough differences can help the partnership be productive later through different perspectives.

A system for matching

By this stage you will have access to information about the mentor's interests and skills (the mentor bio form), and the mentee's needs for support and preferred mentor characteristics (the mentee EOI form). With the information you can narrow down the suitable partnerships. Remember you are looking for something in common to form the basis of the relationship as well as a good fit between mentor offerings and mentee needs. It can be useful to have the information about mentors and mentees listed side by side to make it easier to look for the best fit between mentee wants and mentor offerings.

Using a worksheet, you can put mentee and mentor information side by side, keep track of the partnerships as they form and keep the mentoring workload fairly evenly spread across the mentor group (we suggest no more than five mentees per mentor). An example of a worksheet for this purpose is included in Appendix 2, *Matching worksheet*.

If a mentee does not have any specifications for a mentor, the main matching consideration is how to assign the mentee to a partnership without overloading any mentors.

After the matching is complete, recording the partnerships and the contact details for the mentee and mentor will be useful for later. You will come back to this record over and over through the year. It is worth the initial investment of time.

Introducing the mentor and mentee

Once you have found the closest, or a close enough match that could meet mentee needs, it is time to facilitate the introduction. Email is convenient for communicating with both mentors and mentees the results of the matching process. Be prepared at this stage to receive one or more replies about the match being unsuitable for one reason or another. The email that follows, addressed to the mentee and copied to the mentor, is an example of how an introduction by email can happen.

Dear [Junior Doctor],

Thank you for your expression of interest in being involved in [Mentoring program] as a mentee.

You have been assigned [Mentor] as a mentor for [Year]. Their bio is attached.

You can approach your mentor to discuss your experiences and ideas, ask for feedback, and set and achieve goals. Your mentor is available to listen, provide constructive feedback, and facilitate the progress you have in mind.

As per the charter (attached), this is a strictly confidential service. However there are some exceptions to this. Please see [Website] for details or contact me to discuss for more information in this regard.

Please be in touch with [Mentor] via switch or email. They look forward to hearing from you.

All the best,
[Coordinator]

p.s. If for any reason, this partnership is unsuitable, please let me know and I can make other arrangements for you.

© State of Queensland (Queensland Health) 2011-2013

It is helpful if the mentor contacts the mentee after this email is sent, to introduce themselves and reinforce their availability to the mentee.

Timing

The best time to finalise introductions is during orientation. Early on, the perceived need for mentoring is greatest. Figure 9 shows an example of how matching and introductions can take place over a five-day intern orientation program.

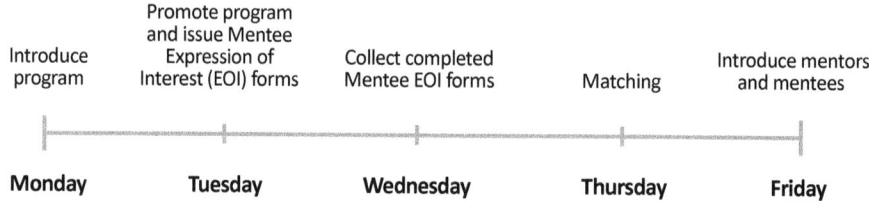

Figure 9. A timeline for completing mentoring partnership formation within a five-day intern orientation program.

You can also encourage a meeting of mentors and mentees soon after the emailed introduction. This meeting can be between one mentor and one mentee, a mentor and their group of mentees, or the whole group of program participants (mentors and mentees). An initial group meeting has a dual purpose of introducing the mentor and mentees and creating an additional opportunity for peer support within the mentee group. This is especially good for new interns who have relocated for internship and are starting out with limited local support networks.

Throughout the year, new mentees can be matched as they apply to the program, and new partnerships can form through mentors referring their mentees to other colleagues for additional support as required.

Further introducing the program

The charter, introduced in Chapter 6, is important as it gives mentees an understanding of what to expect from the program and what the program expects of them. Early in the partnerships, mentors should confirm that the mentees have received and understood the charter.

When the partnership doesn't take off

What if contact does not occur between the mentor and the mentee? Some mentees will not respond to their mentor's emails or other communications, despite the mentor's best intentions and attempts.

If the mentee is not contacting or responding to the mentor, they may lack confidence to do so or have other barriers that can be overcome if the mentor attempts contact later in the year. Alternatively they may wish to be passive participants in the program unless they really need help. An explanation for non-contact may be found on the mentee EOI form if you have included a section about mentees' intended participation levels in the program.

Mentor-initiated contact twice a year reassures mentees of mentors' availability, while respecting the mentees' chosen level of involvement in the program.

Re-matching

Re-matching may be required in certain circumstances, for example if a mentor departs the program or a mentee considers their partnership unsuitable. In these situations, clear and open communication is essential to ensure a satisfactory outcome for all involved.

When a mentor moves on

If a mentor departs the program, give the mentee the option of forming a new partnership with an alternative mentor. The original matching process applies. Check that the proposed new mentor has the intention of being available for the remainder of the year, and introduce the mentor and mentee.

When a partnership is unsuitable

If a mentee considers their partnership unsuitable, a suggested process is to inform the original mentor of the request to change partnerships and the reason for the request. As a courtesy, ask the mentor for their approval to re-assign the mentee. Using the mentee's specifications, identify a suitable match, confirm the proposed mentor's availability and facilitate the introduction.

12. Training 'Ready for Anything' Mentors

Why train mentors?

If mentoring is a partnership and a developmental process, how do you do it? Mentor training answers these questions. Through mentor training, doctors learn to be mentors and to deliver effective mentoring to their mentees.

From the abstract to the actionable

During training, abstract concepts are made actionable, as shown in Figure 10. The partnership concept is converted to the Cycle of Caring (Skovholt, 2005) introduced in Chapter 4. The process is converted to the transformational conversation, with defined elements that can be combined in various ways for purposes such as facilitation or just being there for the mentee.

Mentoring = Partnership (the Cycle of Caring) + Process (transformational conversations)

Figure 10. Making the abstract actionable in mentoring

We cover the transformational conversation in more detail shortly.

A new paradigm of helping

Doctors are trained to listen and ask questions in order to diagnose and problem solve; they are trained to be the expert. Mentors are trained to listen and ask questions in order to understand and facilitate progress important to the mentees; they are trained to let mentees be the expert. Same tools, vastly different applications. A good doctor cannot be a good mentor without understanding the difference in paradigm. Through mentor training, doctors learn to dispense with their usual tools of trade, their scalpels and stethoscopes, and use other tools such as their example, words and presence.

The prepared mentor

The ultimate aim of mentor training is that doctors emerge from training prepared for their role, and 'ready for anything'. Being ready for anything means they are capable of delivering a constructive response, no matter what the issue. This does not contradict the need to have parameters in the mentoring program. If the presenting problem is beyond the scope of a service, an example of a constructive response would be a referral to an appropriate service.

The prepared mentor looks, sounds and acts something like this:

- Looks like – attentive body language, genuine, present
- Sounds like – states availability, has a caring tone, uses listening and silence, questions and informs
- Acts like or is – an ally, a role model, trustworthy, reliable, available, caring toward self and others, responds constructively, facilitates (i.e. makes progress easier).

In this chapter, we focus on design, delivery and evaluation of a group training session for mentors, and offer suggestions for mentors' on-going professional development.

Training design

Adults learn best when the training is relevant to their goals, interests and needs; when the atmosphere is respectful and collaborative; and when the process encourages integration of new content with what they already know.

Learning objectives

Learning objectives give purpose and direction to the training and ideally will link with the needs of the mentors to prepare for their role. The top two content areas for mentor training are:

1. the partnership: how to have a mentoring partnership
2. the process: how to have a transformational conversation, a conversation with the potential to guide, inspire and heal.

Teaching mentoring as a partnership – the Cycle of Caring

All mentoring partnerships have a beginning, a middle and an end, and mentors need to know how to navigate each of these stages. The Cycle of Caring stages of Empathic Attachment, Active Involvement and Felt Separation can be the mentors' guide and the foundation of mentor training.

Teaching mentoring as a process – the transformational conversation

Within the partnership formed by the Cycle of Caring, there could be many conversations. Each conversation has the potential to be transformational, that is to prompt a shift in the mentee from one state of development to another. The three elements of the transformational conversation are:

1. listening
2. questioning
3. informing.

These elements can be mixed and matched for various purposes, including facilitation. Training is an opportunity for mentors to explore how to interweave these conversational elements for facilitation of specific outcomes, such as goal achievement, learning, insight, clinical reasoning and well-being. This will enable their use during mentoring, usually at the Active Involvement stage of the Cycle of Caring. Examples of these transformational conversations are shown in Table 1.

Ensure adequate time is allocated during training for mentors to learn how to facilitate goal achievement and crisis management. Mentors who have facilitation skills in these two areas will be able to provide an initial, constructive response to most mentee issues. Mentors can expand their facilitation repertoire throughout the year by participating in on-going professional development.

An example of training content structured according to the Cycle of Caring is provided in Chapter 18.

Table 1. Examples of transformational conversations: using questioning, listening and informing to facilitate development.

TRANSFORMATIONAL CONVERSATIONS		
Using conversation elements to facilitate...	Facilitation method	Description of the conversation
Goal achievement	GROW (Whitmore, 2009)	GROW is an acronym; each letter stands for a stage and enquiry related to goal achievement. **G – Goal** (desired state) **R – Reality** (current state) **O – Obstacles** (barriers) and options (for overcoming barriers) **W – Way forward** (options are converted to action steps). The mentor takes the mentee through each stage/enquiry until they reach an actionable plan for the way forward.
Reflection	Reflection-on-action (Schon, 1987)	The mentor leads the mentee through enquiries related to what happened in thought and action, and a plan for the way forward, e.g. What happened? What were your actions? What was your thinking related to the actions? What you have you learned that you can take forward with you?
Learning	Clinical teaching (Lake & Ryan, 2004)	The mentor uses questions to establish what the mentee already knows about the topic of interest. This becomes the foundation for new knowledge. After that, the mentor uses questioning and informing to find and fill gaps in the mentee's knowledge.
Clinical reasoning	One Minute Preceptor (Neher, Gordon, Meyer & Stevens, 1992)	The mentor questions and informs the mentee about a clinical care aspect of a case e.g. diagnosis or management, using five microskills: asking for a commitment to a diagnosis or plan, exploring supporting evidence, teaching general rules, verbally reinforcing effective actions, and correcting mistakes.
Well-being	Acceptance and Commitment Therapy (Hayes, 1999)	The mentor uses questions to find a discrepancy between the mentee's values (on-going directions the mentee wishes to take) and the actual directions they are taking, and identifies the thoughts and feelings that may be involved in the discrepancy. The mentor then helps the mentee to manage their thoughts and feelings more effectively through mindfulness so the mentee can be freer to take valued actions.
Stress and crisis management	STOP (Harris, 2007), based on Acceptance and Commitment Therapy	STOP is an acronym; each letter stands for a stage and enquiry related to managing intense emotions and taking helpful, valued action. **S – Slow down.** Slow your breathing; slowly press your feet on the floor, stretch your arms or press your fingertips together. **T – Take note.** With a sense of curiosity, notice your thoughts and feelings, what you can see, hear, touch, taste and smell; notice where you are and what you are doing. **O – Open up.** Make room for your thoughts and feelings and allow them to freely flow through you. **P – Pursue values.** Let your values guide whatever you do next. The mentor talks the mentee through each of these stages, using questions and instructions on where to put their focus.

Competencies

However you decide to describe your learning objectives and structure your content, it is helpful to keep in mind the specific competencies that you would like your mentors to develop. This will ensure that each competency is given sufficient attention during the course of the training. Examples of competencies relevant to mentoring are:

- communicating effectively
- developing a helping partnership
- conducting an initial interview
- assessing risk and managing crises
- facilitating (e.g. goal achievement, learning, insight, clinical reasoning and well-being)
- assessing effectiveness of mentoring
- concluding a mentoring encounter
- concluding a mentoring partnership
- referring on
- practicing self-awareness and self-care
- recording encounters.

Content areas not to miss

Valuable content areas include:

- being a mentor, not a doctor, to mentees
- staging the mentoring partnership according to the Cycle of Caring, using Empathic Attachment, Active Involvement and Felt Separation
- building trust
- forming a mentoring agreement
- structuring a mentoring conversation; using listening, questions and information as mainstays of the transformational conversation
- the empathy statement (i.e. reflecting feeling and content)
- recognising and responding to mentee distress
- a generic and versatile framework for basic facilitation of goal achievement
- the balancing acts of mentors: challenge and support; past, present and future; insight and action; making things easier but not too easy for the mentee
- a mentoring case study

- notifiable conduct by the mentee
- common mentoring challenges
- overcoming challenges
- self-awareness, self-care and mindfulness
- data collection and record-keeping.

A sample training sequence is included in Appendix 2, *Training Run Sheet*.

Customising training based on organisational objectives and priorities

Mentor training is an opportunity to maintain the alignment of the mentor program with organisational objectives and ensure the program not only meets individual mentor learning needs but makes a useful contribution to the organisation's strategic directions. Recognising the organisation's priorities during training also helps to preserve management buy-in and justify continued funding of the program.

Training delivery

Timing of training

Offering training early in the junior doctor year such as Term 1, is ideal, so mentors are prepared for their role from the start. Face-to-face delivery is preferable to allow for experiential learning and interaction as a group. If mentors cannot attend the group training due to clinical commitments, offer them alternative individual options, for example, on-line or self-paced learning.

Venue choice

The best venue for training is somewhere that the mentors can go to distance themselves from their clinical duties and work phones for the duration of training. We like to use a setting that is outdoors in a natural environment with readily available refreshments and nearby facilities. There are many reasons for this choice. Such a location is a distance from work and interruptions. It is a relaxed learning environment. It is a reward to spend time in a setting that is such a contrast to what they usually inhabit. It reminds the mentors that there is a world outside of medicine by day. Finally, it gives them the experience of caring for themselves while caring for others. The mentors tend to leave this type of training ready and refreshed.

Invitation to training

The more notice you give mentors of the upcoming training, the more likely it is they will be able to make arrangements to participate. At the very least, give four weeks' notice. And remember that despite your best efforts to give everyone plenty of notice, things can arise unexpectedly and prevent even the most motivated mentors from attending. That is the nature of hospital life. A sample invitation to training is included in Chapter 14.

Release for training

Enlisting high-level support in authorising the release of mentors for training can help with attendance. The following sample email is from a Deputy Executive Director of Medical Services.

Dear [Supervisor],

[Mentor] has volunteered to be part of the [Mentoring program] that began in [Year], to provide mentoring support for junior doctors in many areas including career direction, work-related issues, and well-being.

All doctors serving as mentors undergo [hours] of training facilitated by the [Unit] at [Hospital]. This will occur on [day, date] from [start time] until [finish time].

This endeavour has the support of the [Executive], [Name].

Could you please ensure [Mentor] is released for this important training? Your help in keeping this program going is greatly appreciated.

Kind regards,

[Deputy Executive Director of Medical Services]
[Hospital]

© State of Queensland (Queensland Health) 2011-2013

Mentor participation

Include your mentors in the delivery of the training content, in order to keep them engaged and to build their confidence and experience in facilitating. This may work by giving them a discussion topic or a scripted experiential learning activity, for example, the trust 'minefield' game, as follows.

We teach trust because it is the foundation of the mentoring relationship. We want mentors to experience the vulnerability of being a mentee, and to decide to be sensitive to that. If mentors have been mentees previously, they get it. We also want the mentors to have an experience of being the mentor to a vulnerable person, and finding ways to be gentle and reassuring when vulnerabilities surface.

The trust game is a good way to do this.

You need a few props here.

The pretend 'minefield' is an area of floor that is littered with obstacles. Any items you have around the place, big or small, will do. You will need to risk manage for this activity and be ready to rescue the mentee if it looks like they will trip. We do not want people tripping in this activity, we just want to simulate the tentativeness they experience as a mentee and the care they take as a mentor. The obstacles on the ground represent the perceived hazards of disclosure as a mentee. The mentee must make their way through the minefield successfully. Here's the catch: they are blindfolded. The mentor is the guide for the mentee. The mentor will guide the mentee through and take care to ensure the mentee stays safe throughout. To get through, the mentee has to take a chance on the mentor's trustworthiness. The mentor has to be trustworthy for this work.

At the end of the game, discuss and describe what it was like for the mentee, and explore what else the mentor could do to alleviate the anxiety of the mentee.

Acknowledging participation

Following the session, issue a certificate to participants to acknowledge their efforts and to verify the training content. An example is provided in Appendix 2, *Certificate of Participation*.

Training evaluation

Training evaluation enables you to assess the effectiveness of the session and improve training for the next group of participants. Sample questionnaires are included in Appendix 2, *Mentor Pre-training Questionnaire* and *Mentor Post-Training Questionnaire*.

After training

The training session is just the start of the process of mentor development. After training, give mentors the opportunity to receive on-going professional development.

Starter kit

A starter kit containing mentoring resources can consolidate mentors' learning and further guide them as they begin to establish mentoring partnerships. The starter kit resources could include a recap of the training session, the chosen approach to mentoring, mentoring competencies, record-keeping resources, and solutions to common mentoring challenges, such as referral points and phone numbers.

Follow-up sessions

Through participation in follow-up sessions, mentors can progress from having basic facilitation skills, for example, skills in facilitating goal achievement, to having advanced facilitation skills, for example skills in facilitating clinical reasoning. A template for scheduling sessions is included in Appendix 2, *Training Calendar*.

The community of practice for on-going professional development

A community of practice is a group of people who share a common interest in a topic, and who come together to share practices and create new knowledge.

A community of practice for mentors is an effective, inclusive and engaging way of up-skilling mentors in mentoring and facilitation techniques, and is a context for learning more about mentoring. It can serve as a regular peer support meeting for mentors to talk about their successes and challenges as mentors, including what has worked and what hasn't during mentoring. It can also serve as a reference group for exploring ideas about the program and potential program changes. A sample lesson plan for a community of practice meeting is included in Appendix 2, *Community of Practice Sample Meeting Plan*.

There are many flexible ways of having a community of practice. It does not always have to be in person. It can be done by email, which is a good way for mentors to stay in touch with each other if they are unable to leave their clinical space and attend meetings.

The usefulness of a community of practice depends on adequate participation by each member of the group, so that there is a sharing and an exchanging between all members, not just a few.

13. Mentoring Service Delivery

The mentoring service delivery dimension of your program is the centerpiece of your program and the core of your program's mission, that is to deliver accessible and relevant mentoring to junior doctors for professional development, career advancement and well-being. All other dimensions of action in the program are in support of mentoring service delivery.

Mentoring service delivery is the domain of the mentors. Through relevant and constructive conversations and other exchanges of communication, mentors keep the program's promise to mentees: the promise of a mentor who is available, trustworthy and relates to them as an ally in their development. The conversations and communication happen within the overarching framework of the partnership, the Cycle of Caring (Skovholt, 2005).

Services

Mentoring by negotiation

How mentoring is delivered is the subject of on-going negotiation between each mentor and mentee. Traditionally, both scheduled conversations, 'coffee shop conversations', and opportunistic conversations, 'corridor conversations', have been the mainstays of mentoring. Contact can also occur by email, phone, or messaging. The aims, activities and frequency of mentoring are also negotiated.

Some mentors choose to have a written agreement with mentees, but most do not. A sample agreement is included in Appendix 2, *Mentoring Agreement template*.

Mentoring on command

A supervisor of a mentee might like to refer a mentee to the program for assistance with developmental needs. The mentoring model we present is designed to foster alliances/mentoring partnerships of two people. The inclusion of a third party can create some complexities that we do not cover in this book. If you do choose to accept referrals from supervisors in your program, ensure there are clear guidelines and shared expectations about how this will work, especially with regards to information-sharing about the mentee.

On-call mentoring

On-call mentoring is an optional extra feature you may like to consider for your program. It can serve several purposes: to cater for junior doctors who want the option of access to advice without being a member of the program, to be an alternative entry point to the program for newly arrived staff to the hospital, and to be a safety net for mentees who need urgent assistance outside their mentor's available times. On-call mentoring relies on a higher level of commitment from mentors because of the significant time, effort and co-ordination required of them to maintain coverage of the on-call service.

Encouraging delivery of mentoring

You can assist mentors in exploring a range of possibilities for supporting their mentee's development. Perhaps the mentors would like to introduce their mentees to other colleagues and networks. They may like to run sessions for their mentees as a group. Find out about each mentor's special interest areas and contributions they could make, such as how to get on to a preferred training program, and check for interest in that topic within the mentee groups. If the interest is there, help your mentors to make it happen. A sample email follows.

> Dear Mentors,
>
> With your help, I'd like to offer the [Year] interns an opportunity to have group mentoring.
>
> If you can spare half an hour in [Month] (anytime that suits you) to run a group discussion (your choice of topic), please let me know by the end of this week.
>
> Kind Regards,
> [Coordinator]
>
> P.S. If you have any other ideas for providing mentoring to doctors attached to [Hospital], please let me know. I can help you with any logistics and planning required.
>
> © State of Queensland (Queensland Health) 2011-2013

Encouraging uptake of mentoring

You can send mentees occasional reminders of the service if you want to help mentors establish or maintain contact with mentees. A sample email follows.

> Dear Doctors,
>
> Thanks for being part of the [Mentoring program] as mentees.
>
> I am writing to encourage you to make contact with your mentor, if you haven't already. Your mentors are willing and able to listen, provide constructive feedback, refer you to resources available, and celebrate your successes.
>
> If you need to be reminded of who your mentor is, or of their contact details, let me know and I'll send you details.
>
> Kind regards,
>
> [Coordinator]
>
> © State of Queensland (Queensland Health) 2011-2013

Mentoring standards

Mentors can adopt a number of standards to guide their mentoring service delivery.

The first standard is the Cycle of Caring (Skovholt, 2005), which relates to the evolution and the focus of the partnership. The three stages of empathic attachment, active involvement and felt separation are milestones that the mentor can use as landmarks during the mentoring process. This keeps mentors on track with progressing the partnership from beginning to middle to end.

A second standard is a 'mentee-centred' approach. Similar to a patient-centred approach, this means the mentor aims to make a difference, as determined by the mentee. This keeps mentoring relevant.

A third standard that can inform mentoring is the Australian Curriculum Framework for Junior Doctors (ACFJD) (http://curriculum.cpmec.org.au). The ACFJD was developed to outline the knowledge, skills and behaviors required of junior doctors. "The Curriculum Framework provides a bridge between undergraduate curricula and the curricula that underpin college training programs. It provides junior doctors with an educational template that clearly identifies the core competencies and capabilities that are required to provide quality health care" (CPMEC, 2006). This can guide priority areas where professional development is the goal of mentoring.

A fourth standard is the mentoring program's charter. It functions as a standard for the values that mentors will enact in their encounters with mentees. It is important for mentors to confirm that the mentees have read and understood the charter, including exceptions to confidentiality and AHPRA's rules about notifiable conduct. Refer to the AHPRA website (www.ahpra.gov.au) for more information.

Finally, we recommend a standard related to the minimum level of outreach by mentors, in recognition of the difficulty that junior doctors may have in asking for help. Ideally, there would be some level of contact each term to coincide with the time that junior doctors are entering new work settings and experiencing new challenges. At a minimum, we suggest that mentors contact mentees at the start of the year to establish or consolidate the partnership, and again halfway through the year to 'check in' with them and remind them of the program.

Monitoring mentoring

Monitoring mentoring involves taking notice of the quality and quantity of mentoring encounters. Monitoring generates information for mentors to use so that they can do more of what works for their mentees. The information is also useful for you to use as coordinator to improve the program during the re-visioning stage of the program.

The *Record of Encounter* (see example provided in Appendix 2) can be a mainstay of monitoring. It is a tool for collecting information about each encounter that takes place within the program, including mentee demographics and reasons for presenting.

A related information collection tool is the *Mentoring Delivery Record*, a service delivery log used by mentors to show overall uptake of mentoring, the amount of time dedicated to mentoring per term, the mode of delivery, and common presentations. An example is provided in Appendix 2.

Both of these records can be used later for evaluation purposes, which we describe in Chapter 17.

Concluding mentoring partnerships

The final act of service delivery is to conclude the mentoring partnerships at the end of the year. This serves a purpose for both mentors and mentees.

For mentees, it clarifies that the mentoring support is concluding and prompts them to put into practice the lessons they have gained from mentoring, such as connectedness, resourcefulness and self-care, and or to find alternative support. For mentors, it acknowledges that they have honoured their commitments and can re-direct their care and concern to others, such as incoming mentees, if they choose to stay on in the program.

This final period can also be a celebration of the developmental journey and achievements of the mentees in partnership with their mentors.

Concluding the mentoring partnerships can be done by the mentors or by you as coordinator. If it is done by mentors, it is the Felt Separation stage of the Cycle of Caring.

The following sample email is from a coordinator.

Dear Doctors,

Thanks for being part of the [Mentoring program] as mentees this year. We hope that your [Year] has been productive and rewarding and that you have found benefit in accessing mentoring.

The program has concluded for the year and the mentoring partnerships are now complete. If you wish to continue on with your mentor, please discuss this with them.

We wish you all the best for the future. Please be in touch if you have any questions.

Kind regards,
[Coordinator] on behalf of [Mentoring program] mentors

© State of Queensland (Queensland Health) 2011-2013

14. Communicating with Mentors

In Chapter 9, we covered communicating with prospective mentors as part of the recruitment process. We now continue our coverage of communicating with mentors, as we look at ways and means of communicating with those who made successful applications.

Why does communicating with mentors matter so much?

Communicating with mentors is purposeful; when used properly, it positively affects their understanding, motivation and actions in relation to the mentoring program.

Sharing understandings

Through communication with mentors, you can establish shared understandings of commitments, agreements and expectations, standards of conduct, and the timing of actions within the program.

Motivating mentors

Providing mentors with feedback about the program improves their motivation and dedication to the task of mentoring. Feedback motivates them to keep doing what they are doing or to make changes in the way they deliver mentoring, if that is indicated. Feedback also shows mentors they are valued.

Influencing mentoring

You will have limited contact with mentees after matching is complete and mentoring commences. Your contact with mentees will be the occasional email of encouragement or information about program opportunities. You are relying on the mentors as a group to deliver a professional service with some consistency across encounters and partnerships. The only way you can influence the quality of mentoring is through your communications with the mentors and the support that you give them.

Reaching mentors

The best methods of communication are the methods that allow you to reach the mentors. For some mentors it may be emails; for some it may be phone calls; for others it may be dropping in at their work space. Emailing all important information enables equitable access to information and a paper trail for record-keeping purposes. Setting up a mailing list with mentors' home and work email addresses takes time initially, but saves a lot of time when used over the course of the year.

In terms of building relationships, personalised emails to individuals and emails to the group of mentors both serve useful purposes. Group emails can help to develop the sense of team within the mentor group. Personalised emails in between group emails can help to maintain relationships between you and individual mentors. Each time you write to mentors, consider the purpose of the communication and which approach fits best.

If you do lose contact with a mentor, it is reasonable to persist in trying various methods of contact to find out if they are still interested in being involved in the program as per their initial commitment.

Within the mentor group you are likely to find one mentor whose motivation and dedication to the cause of junior doctor support is exceptional. This person can take on an unofficial lead mentor role, assisting the coordinator to communicate with mentors between meetings, encouraging participation, and identifying logistical issues from a mentor's point of view.

Reasons to communicate

There are plenty of reasons to keep in touch with the mentors:
- asking for information
- giving information
- issuing invitations
- sending reminders
- showing appreciation.

Asking for information

Throughout the year, you will reach stages and dimensions of implementation that require additional details of or from mentors.

If you need to collect a high volume of information quickly, consider putting the questions into the body of an email (instead of in an attachment) so mentors can reply easily and promptly. When you ask for information, include a deadline so mentors can give your request the prioritisation you would like. The following email text provides an example.

Dear Mentors,

Could you please send me a quick update on your mentoring activity levels since the [Month] training, by [Date] –

1. approx. no. of mentees
2. approx. total hrs of mentoring encounters
3. general description of discussion topic/s, e.g. work performance, work relationships, work-life balance (no identifying information required).

Kind regards,

[Coordinator]

© State of Queensland (Queensland Health) 2011-2013

Giving information

The extent to which mentors become and remain engaged with the program relies somewhat on how much you actively include them in the program and seek out their engagement. Giving out information regularly helps with engagement.

Mentors like to know about:
- program updates
- discussion topics and outcomes of meetings
- support available
- evaluation findings.

Program updates

The mentors' community of practice meetings are opportunities to share and discuss program updates, such as service evolution, service uptake, and how the program is going overall.

Post-meeting follow-ups

Invariably, there will be mentors who are unable to attend meetings and events. Keep them in the loop by providing post-meeting minutes or a brief report, such as below.

Dear Mentors,

I hope your [Year] is off to a good start.

Thanks again for your willingness to be involved in supporting new doctors. We had a record-breaking [Number] requests from interns for mentoring this year.

Here are some details (attached) of the first meeting which took place at [Venue] on [Date, time].

If there is anything you need, please let me know.

Kind regards,

[Coordinator]

© State of Queensland (Queensland Health) 2011-2013

Support available to mentors

Mentors are not immune to the distress of medical practice or feeling the burdens of helping other people, including their mentees. Be prepared for the possibility that you may need to arrange support for a mentor in distress. A designated mentors' mentor is someone who could help a mentor in distress. Alternatively, a Director of Clinical Training could have the ability to act as a resource. If mentor distress is high, a referral to external support may be more appropriate, as per the following example.

> Dear Mentors,
>
> Thanks very much for being part of the [Mentoring program] in [Year] and for being a valuable resource for your junior colleagues. This is to remind you that we appreciate your work with junior doctors and we want to ensure that you are offered the best support for your work. [Doctor] is our designated mentor support person. Please be in touch with [Doctor] if you would like any support for yourself or for your work as mentors. Thanks again for your generosity and goodwill.
>
> Kind regards,
>
> [Coordinator]
>
> © State of Queensland (Queensland Health) 2011-2013

Evaluation findings and change

Ideally, evaluation results are delivered to the mentor group face-to-face, rather than by email, particularly if there is something surprising or contentious within the findings or something that triggers a proposal of change for the program. Exchange of dialogue allows mentors to work together and incorporate various perspectives in understanding and processing the evaluation information.

Issuing invitations

The invitations you will most often issue to mentors are invitations to meetings and training, and at the end of the year, an invitation to continue in the mentor role the following year. Sample emails of invitation follow.

Invitation to a meeting

> Dear Mentors,
>
> Our Term [Term number] meeting will be held on [Date] at [Time], at [Venue]. Minutes will be available after the meeting for those who can't make it. RSVP [Date].
>
> Kind regards,
>
> [Coordinator]
>
> © State of Queensland (Queensland Health) 2011-2013

Invitation to training

> Dear Mentors,
>
> Mentor training will be held on this [Date], at [Venue]. Your participation has been authorised by [Executive] and a letter to verify this is attached for you to give to your supervisor. If you have any trouble gaining permission for training please let us know.
>
> Kind regards,
>
> [Coordinator]
>
> © State of Queensland (Queensland Health) 2011-2013

Invitation to continue in the mentoring role

> Dear Mentors,
>
> Thanks for being part of the [Mentoring program] in [Year] and for being available to your junior colleagues.
>
> As Term [Term number] draws to a close, [Unit] is preparing for the arrival of the [Year] interns and we intend to continue to offer the [Mentoring program] to help new doctors find their way. We would like to invite you to continue in your mentoring role.
>
> Please let me know of your availability by [Date].
>
> Kind regards,
>
> [Coordinator]
>
> © State of Queensland (Queensland Health) 2011-2013

Sending reminders

Remind mentors of actions they have agreed to take, for example, contacting mentees at least twice during the year, as per the following example.

> Dear Mentors,
>
> [Mentor] presented on [Mentoring program] at [Intern Event] today and encouraged mentees to check in with their mentors, so you may hear from them soon. If you haven't heard from them in a while, now is an opportune time for you to make contact with them.
>
> Kind regards,
>
> [Coordinator]
>
> © State of Queensland (Queensland Health) 2011-2013

Showing appreciation

Mentoring service delivery is made possible through the generous contributions of mentors, often in their own time. Show appreciation to mentors for their contributions. Options for conveying appreciation to mentors include a letter of reference, a letter or email of thanks, and a certificate. Sample letters of reference and thanks are shown below, and an example of a certificate is included in Appendix 2, *Recognition of Service Certificate*.

Letter of reference

To whom it may concern,

Re: [Mentor]

I am writing to support [Mentor's] application for training with the [College], in particular to mention their involvement with our hospital's [Mentoring program] since [Date].

The [Mentoring program] offers junior doctors assistance with personal and professional goals. The chosen mentors complete training in assessment, interview techniques, the mentoring role, and psychological support strategies. The program is now in its [Number] successful year here at [Hospital] and has attracted national attention at conferences.

[Mentor] was selected as a mentor on the basis of their commitment to supporting junior doctors and performance and role modelling as a clinician at [Hospital]. They have taken to their role with enthusiasm and dedication. The skills they have acquired in their training for this endeavour, and their positive role modelling, will contribute greatly to their role as a [Specialty] registrar.

Yours sincerely,

[Coordinator or Unit Director, Hospital]

© State of Queensland (Queensland Health) 2011-2013

Letter of thanks

Dear [Mentor],

Thank you for being a mentor of the [Mentoring program] in [Year].

With your help, [Mentoring program] was able to offer mentoring to [Number] junior doctors this year. Following your example of goodwill, [Hospital] has a growing culture of caring for each other, with [Number] new mentors stepping up to follow your lead.

A certificate of appreciation from [Executive] is to follow.

I wish you all the best for the future.

Kind regards,

[Coordinator]

© State of Queensland (Queensland Health) 2011-2013

Communications schedule

When do these communications take place? The timing and volume of communication varies from program to program and depends on the need for exchanges of information. Here are some suggestions for the timing of essential communications across the 5-term junior doctor year (January to January) after the initial recruitment and orientation of mentors is complete.

Term 1: Notice of partnerships, invitation to first meeting, post-meeting follow-up, invitation to training.

Terms 2, 3 and 4: Invitation to community of practice meeting, post-meeting follow-up.

Term 5: Invitation to community of practice meeting, post-meeting follow-up, request for mentoring delivery data and mentor feedback, notice of intention to conclude mentoring partnerships, release of evaluation results, invitation to return as mentors the following year, letter and certificate of appreciation.

15. Information Management

Your program is a generator of information, stemming from communication between mentors and mentees, and communication between you and your program's stakeholders. The information will consist of program information and personal information. You, as the coordinator, are the program's information manager. For program information, your information management goals are distribution, filing and archiving. For personal information, your goals are purposeful use, privacy, confidentiality and access to records.

This chapter focuses on the management of personal information. We offer general guidelines for collecting, using, storing and disclosing personal information. Personal information management is governed by laws pertaining to privacy, confidentiality and access to records, so it is essential that you are familiar with current commonwealth and state legislation. Keep in mind that laws vary from state to state, and organisational guidelines can add further variations. We encourage you to seek legal advice prior to implementing information management.

What is personal information?

> Personal information is information or an opinion, including information or an opinion forming part of a database, whether true or not, and whether recorded in material form or not, about an individual whose identity is apparent, or can be reasonably ascertained, from the information or purpose (Office of the Information Commissioner Queensland, 2012).

Information is personal information if it is about an individual and it allows the individual's identity to be ascertained from the information itself or from cross-referencing with other information.

Examples of personal information are an individual's:

- name
- address
- phone number
- photo
- education.

Personal information can also be sensitive information. Sensitive information includes information about an individual's health, membership of a professional association, cultural background, religious and philosophical beliefs, and political opinions.

Sources of personal information in a junior doctor mentoring program

The two main sources of personal information in a junior doctor mentoring program are the mentor and mentee applications to join the program, and the mentoring conversations between mentors and mentees.

Mentee and mentor applications

To make an application to the program, mentees and mentors supply personal information, for example, their name and contact details. With this information, you can form partnerships, make introductions, and maintain contact with each participant. Examples of application paperwork are the mentor nomination described in Chapter 9 and the Mentee EOI form introduced in Chapter 10.

Mentor and mentee disclosures

Disclosures by mentees and mentors are an essential part of mentoring. Mentees may find out things about their mentor's past or current circumstances as part of the sharing of experience provided by the mentor. Mentors will find out all sorts of things about their mentees: their past challenges and accomplishments, their present personal and professional circumstances, and their future plans, such as for streaming or promotion. You too may come across clues about mentees as you collect information to monitor and evaluate the program.

Communicating expectations about personal information management

All program participants need to understand and commit to personal information management practices for confidentiality, privacy and access to records. As a rule, all information is treated as confidential, or the level of confidentiality is discussed and agreed. When personal information management practices are clearly defined, the program feels safe to participants. Two ways to formally communicate your program's expectations about personal information management practices are the program charter and the confidentiality agreement, introduced in Chapters 6 and 9 respectively.

The charter

The charter outlines the program's and the mentors' promises to mentees. It also explains the rights and responsibilities of mentors and mentees in regards to personal information management, particularly confidentiality. An example of a charter is provided in Chapter 18.

The confidentiality agreement

A confidentiality agreement is a written agreement between the program and the mentors, presented as a condition of participating in the program. The agreement is confirmation that the mentors understand the need for confidentiality, the limits to confidentiality and the consequences of breaching confidentiality.

Collecting information

Before collecting personal information from program participants, let participants know how their information will be used, who will have access to their information, and their right to access their information. Do not collect sensitive information without the participants' consent.

Mentors do not have to keep mentoring records. There is no legal requirement for them to do so. They may prefer for mentees to keep their own mentoring records or a mentoring journal if desired. We encourage you to seek legal advice about the advantages and disadvantages of record-keeping by mentors in your program.

Using information

Information that is collected should be used for the purposes specified during collection. For you as the coordinator, the purposes will be partnership formation, introductions and communications with program participants. For the mentors, the purposes will be communication with mentees and support for mentees' development. Information may also be used to prevent harm to another, as we will explain shortly.

Storing information

You will need a filing system for records of current participants and an archiving system for records of past participants, as well as a plan for when and how to destroy records. All records must be stored securely, with access restricted to those who were identified during collection as requiring the information. For hard copy records, use a secure filing system. For electronic records, use a password-protected file, with a plan in place for periodic back up of the file.

If mentors choose to keep written records of their mentoring, they may like to use a coding system as a confidentiality measure. An example of a coding system is extracting the identifying information and using a numerical or alphabetical code on the record, while storing the corresponding identifying information in a separate database.

Disclosing information

While much of the information provided is generally confidential in nature there are circumstances where this information may still be disclosed to a third party. For example:

- where there is a duty of care to do so
- where notifiable conduct has occurred
- where a court has made an order for the information to be disclosed
- an individual has made a request for access to the information.

Duty of care

Duty of care is the duty to take reasonable care to prevent another being harmed. It involves identifying a likely risk of harm, and taking reasonable care in response.

For example, if a mentee has made serious threats of harm to him or herself or others, it is appropriate for the mentor to disclose this information to a third party, such as a Crisis Assessment and Treatment Team (CATT), police or family, for intervention. Where possible, the mentor should inform the mentee in advance that they will be disclosing information and explain why.

Notifiable conduct

Notifiable conduct refers to behaviours by health practitioners registered with the Australian Health Practitioner Regulation Agency (APHRA) that trigger mandatory notification to AHPRA. The behaviours are:

- practicing under the influence of alcohol or drugs
- sexual misconduct
- impairment affecting work performance and creating risk
- departing from acceptable professional standards.

No one likes to talk about the reporting of notifiable conduct in relation to a mentoring program because it has the potential to destabilize a program and cast doubt upon its reliability as a trustworthy service. But it is so important that it needs some emphasis. From the start of the program's relationship with mentees, ensure all mentees are made aware that notifiable conduct must, by law, be reported.

Refer to the website of the Australian Health Practitioner Regulation Agency (AHPRA) (www.ahpra.gov.au) for more details on reporting notifiable conduct.

Court orders

A court may order that confidential information is to be disclosed. For example a court may require disclosure in response to a witness summons or a subpoena to produce documents.

It is important to note that the requirements of courts with regards to the disclosure of confidential information may vary from state to state. As such it is strongly recommended that you seek legal advice prior to the disclosure of any information which you believe to be confidential.

Requests for access

Program participants can have access to their records on request. If an agency requests information about a program participant, obtain the participant's consent in writing prior to the release of records.

16. Maintaining the Program's Profile

Maintaining the program's profile is about promoting awareness and understanding of the program among stakeholders and the community for the duration of the program.

Why maintain the program's profile?

Encouraging participation by mentors and mentees

Program information can remind mentors and mentees to make time for mentoring in their busy schedules, and engage them in new opportunities to participate in the program.

Introducing the program to new doctors

New medical staff join hospitals throughout the year and appreciate access to information about programs and services available to them. If information is delivered infrequently or only at the start of the year, incoming staff, who may be within your target groups of mentors and mentees, may miss out on receiving the information and on the opportunity to be involved.

Recognising and celebrating the contributions of mentors

Keeping the profile of the program high recognises the contributions of mentors. This acknowledgement and valuing of mentors can gain the attention of aspiring mentor applicants and influence them to apply.

Sponsorship success

Visibility of a mentoring program helps sponsors when making funding decisions and can enhance the program's prospects of receiving continuing funding and organisational support.

Making a statement for cultural change

An underlying reason to maintain a mentoring program's profile relates to de-stigmatising junior doctors' access to care. As we have considered in Chapter 4, a mentoring program is not just about delivering mentoring, it is also about making a clear statement that conversation is helpful, connectedness is healthy, and effective other-care relies on sufficient self-care. A high-profile program can do some of the work of making these statements and contributing to cultural change.

Options for maintaining your program's profile

Newsletters

Many hospitals produce and issue a newsletter on a regular basis and accept submission of stories or advertisements for inclusion. Consider requesting a feature of your mentoring program, or recruitment advertisements for mentors or mentees, in the newsletter.

Media

Be newsworthy and get your program in the news if you can. Your hospital may have a public relations coordinator with experience in writing press releases to attract media attention. A program launch is an activity that often interests the media.

Posters

Posters can be used to introduce the program, clarify what is on offer through the program, introduce the mentors, and provide instructions for joining the program as a mentee or for contacting mentors. Consider the following tips for producing and displaying posters:

- Have an attention-grabbing headline.
- Ask the mentors to provide the content for the poster - it is a fairly public display of their personal information and they need to decide how much they are comfortable revealing about themselves in this way.
- Include what mentors do and what mentees do in a mentoring partnership.
- Do not display these in public areas, such as hospital walkways and patient care areas.

Mentor program badges

Issued to mentors, mentor program badges can serve many purposes. They help to identify mentors, contribute to the sense of team, and start conversations. For some, a badge is also a reward. If you choose to use badges for these purposes, we suggest you choose ones that can easily be attached to a lanyard and are the correct size, are durable, and are a suitable design that mentors like.

Website

Giving the program an online presence allows stakeholders to have immediate access to the latest program information.

Professional forums

Agencies that care about support for junior doctors are likely to be interested in your program and may encourage you to deliver presentations. For example, state and national medical education forums are often interested in featuring presentations about junior doctor support, either through poster presentations or speaking engagements. Gaining visibility in this way can also benefit your program by creating connections and opportunities to share ideas with programs at other sites. You may also find avenues for submitting articles on your program to various professional journals.

Networking events

Networking events bring program participants together. Advertising and offering networking events raises awareness of the program, generates interest, and provides mentors and mentees with a space for establishing and strengthening mentoring partnerships in a relaxed group session.

17. Evaluating the Program

What is program evaluation?

Program evaluation is a purposeful set of activities for increasing the understanding of one or more aspects of your program. The essential activities of evaluation are deciding on the purpose of the evaluation, forming questions, collecting data, analysing data, interpreting the results, and reporting on findings.

Evaluation has many uses:

- Monitoring, to ensure the program design is implemented as planned and mentoring is reaching the target group. Monitoring includes keeping track of the resources going into the program, the activities taking place, and the direct products of the activities, as well as describing the characteristics of the program and its context.
- Improving, to make the program the best it can be. When completed, evaluation allows you to carry out re-visioning, the culminating step of program development. Re-visioning is a design review process for preparing for the next year of the program. It involves checking the relevance of the program's vision and mission for the way forward and deciding to continue the program as is, continue with adjustments, or discontinue the program. Evaluation gives you a basis for this decision-making.
- Generating effective program designs. Evaluation of many programs can generate effective designs or models that identify which activities generally lead to the best outcomes and how variations in programs affect outcomes.
- Accountability, to justify to sponsors and other stakeholders the resourcing of the program.
(Centres for Disease Control and Prevention, 2008)

In this chapter, we look at mentoring program evaluation using two complementary types of evaluation: process evaluation and outcome evaluation. But first, we look at how evaluation fits within the Mentoring Program Development Model.

Evaluation in the Mentoring Program Development Model

Within the Mentoring Program Development Model, evaluation is carefully planned before it is implemented, as highlighted in Figure 11. The importance of planning an evaluation relates to the need to factor in the interests and agendas of diverse stakeholders, to collect data at specific times during the program, and to ensure approval by the Human Research Ethics Committee (HREC) if required prior to evaluating. Refer to the HREC website (www.nhmrc.gov.au) for more information.

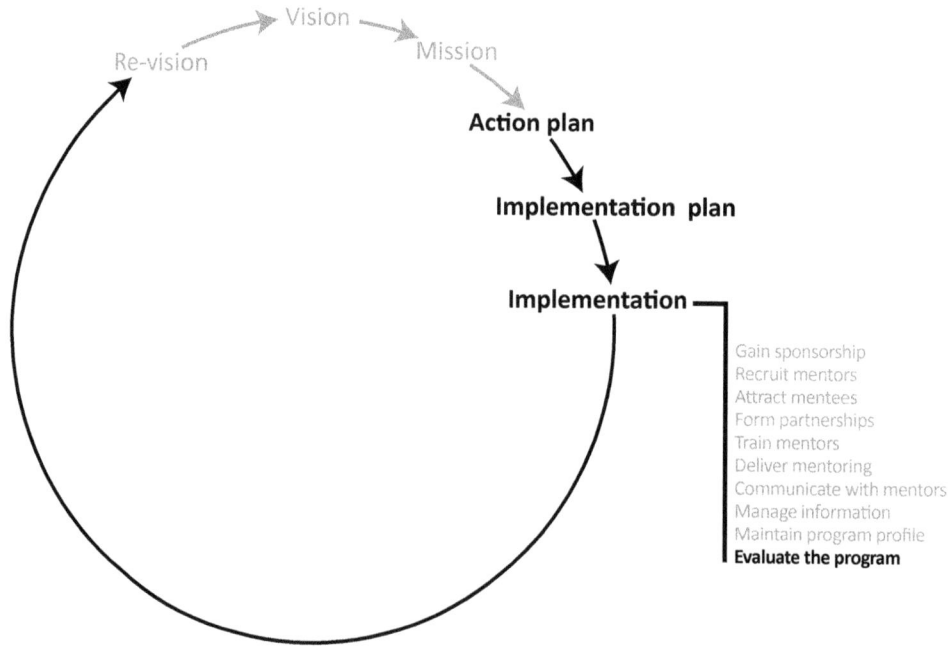

Figure 11. The necessity of evaluation planning prior to evaluation implementation.

Evaluation planning

Evaluation planning involves deciding on the purpose of the evaluation, the questions you will answer, what you will measure, data collection and analysis methods you will use, who will perform each evaluation activity, what will happen with the information, and how you will share your findings.

Ethical considerations

Research that involves contact with human subjects usually requires Human Research Ethics Committee (HREC) review to ensure the research is conducted in an ethical way. An activity where the primary purpose is to monitor or improve quality of service, such as program evaluation, is a quality assurance (QA) activity. Many QA and evaluation activities require oversight but do not require ethical review. According to the National Health and Medical Research Council:

> Irrespective of whether an activity is QA, evaluation or research, the activity must be conducted in a way that is ethical. This should include consideration of whether the people involved will be exposed to any harm as a result of the activity. Those conducting the activity need to consider a range of issues including consent, privacy, relevant legislation, national/professional standards, and whether ethical review is required (NHMRC, 2014).

Refer to *Ethical considerations in quality assurance and evaluation activities* (NHMRC, 2014) for further information about appropriate oversight of program evaluation and for guidance on when an ethical review is required.

Evaluation implementation

Data collection is carried out continuously through the year, with data analysis, interpretation, and reporting typically occurring at the end of the implementation phase towards the end of the junior doctor year.

Process and outcome evaluations

A complete program evaluation comprises a process evaluation used in conjunction with an outcome evaluation. These two types of evaluations require the same activities, that is deciding on the purpose of the evaluation, forming questions, collecting data, analysing data, interpreting the results, and reporting on findings, but have a very different focus. We will cover each evaluation separately, and then explain their combined use for a comprehensive mentoring program evaluation.

Process evaluation

The focus of a process evaluation is on describing a program and how it functions over time, as well as the context of the program.

According to Centers for Disease Control and Prevention (2008) and MacDonald et al. (2001), three types of related information are central to describing a program: inputs, activities and outputs. Inputs are the financial, material and human resources invested in the program, activities are processes that generate the program's services and products, and outputs are services and products that the program provides. In a mentoring program, inputs include staff and funds, activities are processes for engaging and preparing mentors and mentees, and outputs are mentoring services.

Contextual information relevant to a process evaluation includes the developmental stage of the program and the environment in which the program exists, for example the current political, social and economic conditions potentially affecting the program design, implementation and accessibility.

The rationale for the process evaluation is that it allows you an understanding of what took place in and around the program. It also reveals any discrepancies between the design and the implementation of the program (CDC, 2008). The process evaluation gives you the story behind the program results.

Process indicators related to input, activity and output

Process indicators are the specific, observable measures of inputs, activities and outputs used in a process evaluation. For a junior doctor mentoring program these can include the following.

Inputs:
- number of mentors
- ratio of male to female mentors
- hours of coordinator time
- seniority/postgraduate year of mentors
- total cost of the program.

Activities:

- number of mentor meetings held
- number of networking events organised
- hours of mentor training delivered
- timing of introductions
- occasions of mentor-initiated contact.

Outputs:

- hours of mentoring conversations
- number of mentoring partnerships
- percentage of mentoring partnerships that are active
- Cycle of Caring approach to mentoring
- perceived suitability of the mentoring partnerships.

Process information on its own is neutral, and remains purely descriptive until you establish standards to compare it with. This is where the results measurements from your implementation plan are relevant and useful. These provide standards for comparison with your program's process indicators.

Outcome evaluation

The focus of an outcome evaluation is on identifying effects of a program's outputs. In a mentoring program, the outcome evaluation explores the effect of the mentoring on mentees and whether it brought about the intended changes, for example, junior doctor development and well-being.

For an outcome evaluation, the two main types of research design are:

1. experimental design (with or without a control group)
2. observational design (e.g., case report, case series, cross-sectional study, or longitudinal study).

An experimental design is generally the strongest design for establishing a cause-effect relationship (Berg & Latin 2011). There are several different types of experimental designs that are appropriate for outcome evaluation. In this setting, the most basic experimental design is a pre/post study (or before and after study) which refers to those studies where measurement(s) are taken before the program implementation, and then the same measurements are repeated after the program has been implemented. This allows measurement of any changes that have occurred due to the program. However, it can be difficult to attribute any observed changes solely to the program, in the absence of a control group. There may be some other explanation for the observed changes, such as a change in hospital protocol, work hours, or staffing. Thus, experimental designs which employ a control group are considered superior (Berg & Latin 2007; Webb & Bain 2011; Kumar 2010). A randomised controlled study is generally considered the strongest design (Berg & Latin 2007; Webb & Bain 2011), but is also the least feasible in this setting. A non-randomised controlled trial is an alternative, but again, less feasible than a pre/post study in this setting.

Outcome indicators

Outcome indicators are the specific, observable measures of outcomes used in an outcome evaluation. For a junior doctor mentoring program these can include:

- application of learning
- levels of stress or distress
- goal achievement
- mid-term appraisal results
- end-of-term assessment results
- a successful application to a training program
- the number of mentees applying to become mentors.

The outcome evaluation can give you the program results, but not the story behind the results.

Why use process evaluation in conjunction with outcome evaluation?

When used together, a process evaluation and an outcome evaluation can provide the fullest understanding of your program: the program results and the story behind the results. By combining process and outcome evaluations, you can make a link between program inputs, activities and outputs, and outcomes. You can also show the optimal path for achieving a specific result and identify ways to improve the program's effectiveness (CDC, 2008; MacDonald et al., 2001). The combined process evaluation and outcome evaluation sequence is shown in Figure 12.

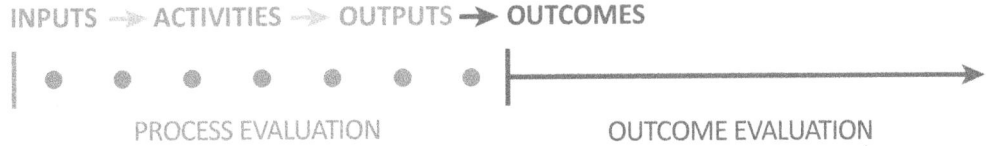

Figure 12. Combining the process and outcome evaluations for a comprehensive program evaluation.
Source: Adapted from Centers for Disease Control and Prevention (2001 & 2008).

When mentoring is effective in supporting junior doctor development and well-being, the process and outcome evaluation shows the inputs, activities and outputs that lead to this result. The sequence is illustrated with an example in Figure 13.

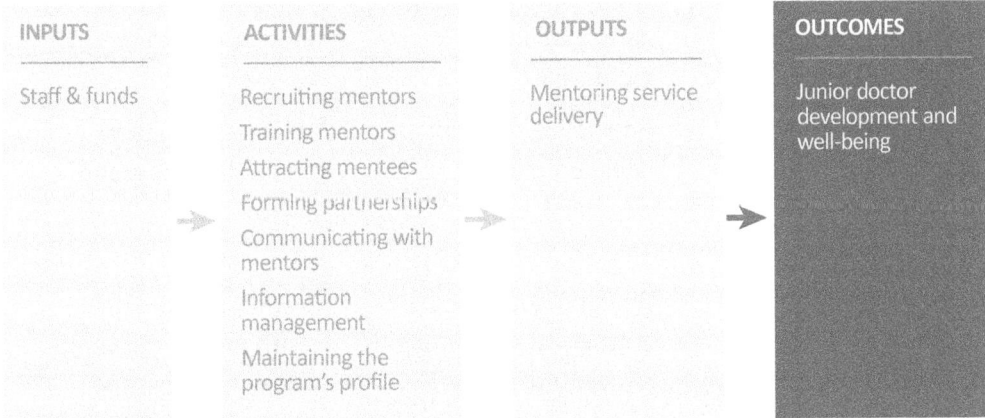

Figure 13. The process and outcome evaluation in context.

Forming questions

What do you want to know about your program's processes and outcomes? The questions you ask will depend on the purpose of your evaluation, and your stakeholders' needs for information and answers.

Process evaluation questions

Process evaluation questions relate to inputs, activities and outputs. Examples are listed in Table 2.

Table 2. Examples of process evaluation questions related to program inputs, activities and outputs.

PROCESS EVALUATION QUESTIONS		
Input	**Activity**	**Output**
What is the total amount we spend on this program?	How do we communicate expectations within the program?	How many partnerships are there?
What resources do we provide to mentors?	What training is offered to mentors?	What percentage of mentoring partnerships is active?
What is the seniority/ postgraduate year of the mentors?	How does the coordinator encourage participation in mentoring?	What are the demographics of the mentees we reach?
How many hours per week does the coordinator work on and in the program?	How is the program being promoted?	Are we reaching the intended target group?
How many of the new mentors have prior mentoring experience?	What on-going support is provided to mentors to carry out their role?	How many hours of mentoring are delivered each term across the program?

Outcome evaluation questions

Outcome evaluation questions relate to changes that occurred because of the program, for example:

- What goals did mentees achieve as a result of mentoring?
- What was the impact of mentoring on mentees' stress levels?
- What were the unintended outcomes of the mentoring program?
- How did the mentoring program change the work environment?
- How did the mentoring program change the mentees' patient care?

In a program dedicated to providing relevant support to many mentees, the goals of each mentee will be diverse, and the outcome evaluation should be able to capture the breadth of changes mentees experience.

Process and outcome questions based on the Kirkpatrick Model

The Kirkpatrick Model (Kirkpatrick, 1967) is a model for evaluating the impact of educational experiences. It applies to mentoring programs for junior doctors because mentoring is a type of educational experience. The Kirkpatrick Model combines aspects of process evaluation and outcome evaluation over four levels, as follows.

Level 1: Reaction
Level 2: Learning
Level 3: Behaviour
Level 4: Results

The questions you form can be based on these levels. For example,

Level 1: Reaction.
Are mentees and mentors satisfied with their experience and did they like being part of the program?

Level 2: Learning.
Did mentees increase their knowledge and or skills through the program?

Level 3: Behaviour.
Did mentees apply any of the knowledge that they learned, i.e. did they take action based on their learning?

Level 4: Results.
What impacts did the mentoring program have on the organisation or society?

Collecting data

Evaluation data can be quantitative (numerical, for quantifying aspects of the program) and qualitative (narrative, for understanding the experience of those involved). The data you need will depend on the questions you are seeking to answer. You may need to develop data collection instruments to collect the data you need.

The mentors' role in data collection

Mentors can help you to collect evaluation information and gauge mentee satisfaction informally throughout the year. You will rely on them for this information if you have limited contact with mentees after matching is complete. Gather this information from mentors periodically to build your data set for the program evaluation at the end of the year. This will allow assessment of changes over time. Data collection should be made as easy as possible for the mentors otherwise they may be reluctant to participate in data collection.

End-of-year data collection

Ideally, some data will be collected at the beginning of the year (before the program begin), and at the end of the year, with further data being collected directly from mentees. Where possible, collect the data yourself, so mentors can keep the focus on the mentoring and the needs of the mentees. Mentees are more likely to tell you if they are unhappy with the service, than to tell the mentor directly. Also collect information from mentors, about mentors. Pencil and paper forms, and surveys by email or Survey Monkey, are simple ways to collect data. Refer to the Survey Monkey website (www.surveymonkey.com) for more information.

Sources of data

Your main data sources for evaluation are the surveys which you administer to mentees and mentors, mentoring records and informal conversations with program participants.

Surveys

Surveys give mentors and mentees the opportunity to reflect on their experiences of the program and their attitudes towards the program, and to generate qualitative and quantitative data. For example:

- Mentor Experience Questionnaire – Explores various aspects of the mentor's experience of the program including suitability of the match, rewards of participation, and attitude towards the program; it also explores the mentor's experience of the adequacy, accessibility, and usefulness of the training and support provided.

- Mentee Experience Questionnaire – Explores various aspects of the mentee's experience of the program, including suitability of the match, benefits of participation, and attitude towards the program.

Sample questionnaires are included in Appendix 2, *Mentor Experience Questionnaire* and *Mentee Experience Questionnaire*.

Records

Records can be useful tools for collection and storage of largely quantitative data. For example:

- Record of Encounter – Shows who the mentees are (gender and postgraduate year), and when, how, and why they participated in mentoring.
- Mentoring Delivery Record – Shows the quantity of mentoring delivered by a mentor each term (and consequently the mentoring uptake trends across the year), the method of delivery, and the mentees' reasons for presenting. This is a compilation by each mentor of their Records of Encounter.
- Coordinator's Annual Mentoring Delivery Log – Shows the total mentoring delivery within the program, across the year and across partnerships, as well as the variety of reasons mentees sought mentoring. This is a compilation by the coordinator of the Mentoring Delivery Records of all the mentors.

Templates are included in Appendix 2, *Record of Encounter*, *Mentoring Delivery Record* and *Coordinator's Annual Mentoring Delivery Log*.

Conversations

Your conversations and catch-ups with mentors, and occasionally mentees, can also be rich sources of qualitative and quantitative data about demand for mentoring, participant (mentor and mentee) satisfaction, and mentee gains.

Mentors can gauge mentee gains and satisfaction during each mentoring encounter. A simple question such as "Was this helpful for you?" can yield useful, usable information for evaluation.

Use a system that works for you to collect and manage your assorted data throughout the year. It is important that you collect the information within and between mentors and mentees in a consistent manner. While conversations can be a useful source of information, it is crucial that they are well documented to avoid measurement error. This can be achieved by using notes, recording the conversations (with prior permission of course), using a semi-structured interview (for example, ensuring that certain topics are covered or questions are asked) when conversing, a more structured approach where a bank of questions are referred to, or describing the conversation using a template (Kumar, 2010; Berg & Latin, 2007).

Collecting with care

The upside of evaluating a junior doctor mentoring program is finding evidence of value. Sponsors appreciate it and need it. The downsides of evaluation for a junior doctor mentoring program are that evaluation data collection can take up valuable mentor time, interfere with the flow of a session, distract from the work of mentoring, and take the focus off the mentee's needs and reasons for presenting.

Collect data as infrequently as possible, do it as unobtrusively as possible, and only measure what you intend to act on. Tell the participants what you will do with the data and findings, and do what you pledge to do in order to preserve trust.

Analysing the data and interpreting the results

Your analysis of data will depend both on your research design and the data which you have collected. If you are using a non-experimental design such as a case study, collate and describe your data for each indicator of inputs, activities, outputs and outcomes. If you are using an experimental design such as pre/post study, quantitative data will be expressed in statistical terms, for example, descriptive statistics such as means, medians, or percents. If any change has been measured, use the appropriate statistic to describe the magnitude of change (t-test; ANOVA; chi-squared test), and the extent to which chance is a possible explanation for the observed change (p-value; 95% Confidence Interval) (Berg & Latin, 2007; Triola & Triola, 2013). It is important to remember that for quantitative data, the number of participants will also impact on the validity of the results, and any consequent interpretations (Triola & Triola, 2013). Qualitative data will be organised into common themes. For the process indicators, compare your indicators with your results measures specified in your implementation plan. For the outcomes indicators, develop an argument for the theoretical link between the intervention and the effect, showing where possible that there is no alternative explanation for the observed changes. Also give consideration to how contextual factors may have impacted on your results.

Decoding the numbers

Interpretation will always involve some subjectivity. Some possible interpretations of findings include:

- high number of mentee EOIs = interest in the program, appeal of the program to mentees, prominent program profile, number of people with intention to have mentoring or a safety net, perceived safety of the service, trust in the program, peer group pressure
- high number of new mentor applications = interest in the program and appeal of the program to prospective mentors
- high number of returning mentor applications = rewards of the program to mentors
- high number of mentees applying to be mentors = satisfaction with the program and commitment to passing on the sharing of expertise
- high number of mentoring hours = desire for service, satisfaction with the service
- number of requests for a mentor = popularity of mentor, reputation of mentor
- number of partnerships formed = number of safety nets but not necessarily the amount of mentoring
- number of inactive partnerships = discomfort and unfamiliarity as a barrier to participation. Counter-intuitively, little or no uptake of services could also mean the safety net is working and doctors are being reassured, to the extent that they do not need further assistance (just knowing a mentor is there is reassuring, so not using the program could be a positive).

Ideally, your data analysis and interpretation will answer the questions which you formed at the start of the evaluation process.

Your definition of success

Ultimately, you are seeking an understanding of how well your program performed in relation to your definition of success. What is your definition of success? Consider how success would look for your program in terms of process and outcome evaluation results. Within your data set, look for evidence of your version of success. Also consider success shortfalls, that is, significant discrepancies between your definition of success and the evaluation results. In what areas of your program were there success shortfalls? As part of the re-visioning process, these success shortfalls can become your priority areas for improvement in the next year of the program.

After evaluation

What do you do with evaluation results? Do something! You build trust with participants by acting on the results, especially if concerns have been raised during the evaluation process. The main categories of action are to continue the program as is, continue the program with adjustments, or discontinue the program.

Some adjustments could be:

- creating targeted interventions in response to prevalent or systemic issues
- adding new mentoring activities
- incorporating new ways of delivering mentoring
- recruiting more mentors
- offering mentors more training or support
- increasing advertising of the program.

Reporting on findings

Reporting to the sponsor

Report back to the sponsor each year to demonstrate the return on their investment. Whatever evidence you have of the program's value, such as process and outcome evaluations results, belongs in that report. Include information about any limitations of the evaluation. Your report will also be of interest to other stakeholders who have supported your program, for example the mentors, the mentors' mentor, and the unit director.

A report template is provided in Appendix 2, *Annual Report template*. The format incorporates the two focal points of evaluation: process and outcomes including questions asked and answered, and a section for an overall interpretation of results in light of your definition of success, as well as recommendations for the way forward.

Reporting to new mentors

Do not let lessons learned go to waste. Consider forming new guidelines based on evaluation results and share these with new mentors, so that they can learn from the past and move forward with what works, and discarding what has not. For example, a mentee may report that they had an encounter with a mentor in which they disclosed a high amount of distress and would have liked follow-up from the mentor. The lesson here, and a possible new guideline, is that mentor follow-up with a mentee may be helpful if mentee distress is high.

A continuously improving cycle

With evaluation complete, you return to the design phase to carry out re-visioning, the culminating step of program development, as shown in Figure 14. By incorporating evaluation findings into re-visioning, you can start the next year of the program with a renewed, progressive design that reflects the current needs of the target group and fits with the program's environment.

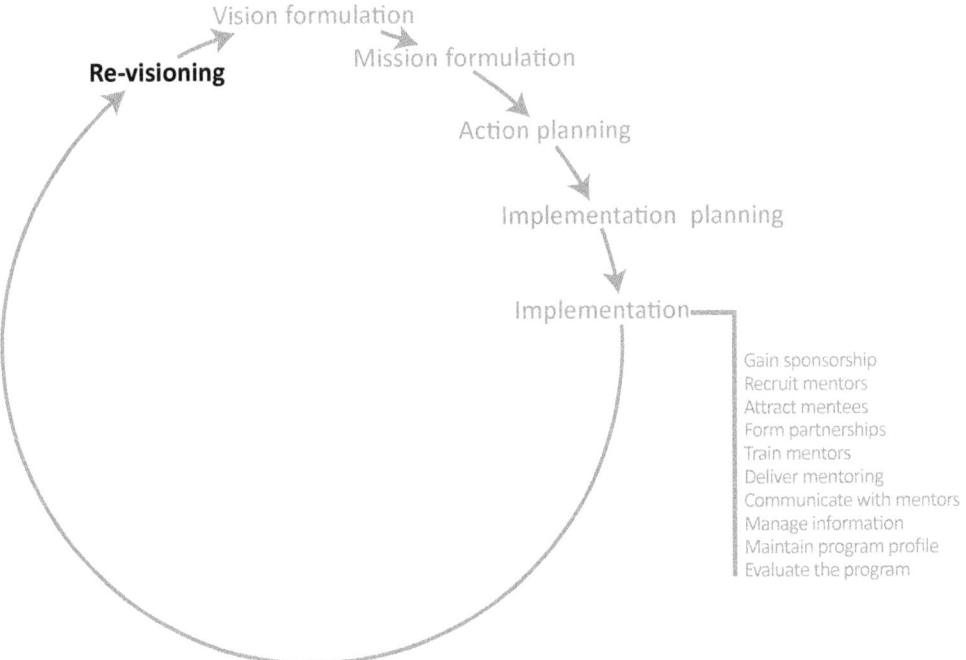

Figure 14. The Mentoring Program Development Model, with a focus on re-visioning.

The complete cycle of mentoring program design and implementation is illustrated in Part Four, which offers a case study of The Townsville Hospital's Doctors for Doctors. It includes program history, design, implementation, lessons learned, and mentors and their stories.

4 Part Four:
The Townsville Hospital Experience

18. The Doctors for Doctors Mentoring Program

History of Doctors for Doctors

We founded Doctors for Doctors at The Townsville Hospital in 2011. The Postgraduate Medical Education Unit (PGMEU), its oversight committee, the General Clinical Education Committee (GCEC), and the Executive Director of Medical Services (EDMS) agreed that a mentoring program could make a unique contribution to supporting interns during their transition from medical school to the workforce, and approved the program for launch.

An enthusiastic team of doctors was recruited as the program's founding mentors. Advertising of the mentor positions occurred via a number of channels including email and posters, which explained the program's initiatives and invited interested doctors to apply by submitting a short biography, an overview of their interests, and strengths the applicant could bring to the program. The final selection of mentors was completed by the PGMEU and the Director of Clinical Training (DCT) to ensure a fair process.

Following recruitment, the founding mentors participated in the design phase of the program. Soon after, the launch of the program was celebrated with an event and media coverage by the local newspaper and the hospital newsletter.

Initially, the program began with a focus on well-being. It soon became apparent that interns were not comfortable with the idea of joining a program that drew attention to their vulnerabilities. During the year, the program was re-branded as an initiative focusing on career development, professional support and guidance. An on-call mentor roster was trialled to provide rapid access to the program's mentors. This was discontinued after no requests for urgent assistance were received.

Support and training for mentors was a major focus of the program and through surveying the mentors, a valuable byproduct of the program was recognised. From the training provided, mentors were developing skills that they could apply outside of mentoring partnerships, in their interactions with patients and in their personal lives.

The original design did not include matching mentors with mentees, and in its first year, 2011, there was no uptake of mentoring services. In 2012, a matching process for partnership formation was initiated and forty-seven percent of interns requested a mentor.

By 2013, the importance of timing was recognised. Introducing the program during the early stages of orientation week created high levels of interest in the program. Eighty-three percent of interns requested a mentor.

PGMEU continues to offer Doctors for Doctors as a key component of its Intern Education and Training Program (IETP).

Mentors and mentees

Mentors are current employees of The Townsville Hospital who have successfully completed at least one year of work at The Townsville Hospital, and who are interested in helping their junior peers to make the transition from medical school to the workforce. Mentors are up to Registrar level of seniority.

Mentees are interns who are new to The Townsville Hospital. Newly arrived International medical graduates are also welcome to access mentoring through the program.

All mentors and mentees participate voluntarily in the program.

The Doctors for Doctors design

Vision, mission and charter

The program's vision is resourceful, resilient and effective junior doctors. The mission of the program is to deliver accessible, relevant mentoring to interns for professional development, career advancement and well-being. The charter is the extended mission, and is shown in Figure 14. The charter explains what interns can expect from the program and what the program expects from them. It also explains the option to give feedback about the program.

Doctors for Doctors Charter

We are committed to providing junior doctors with accessible and meaningful support. Our Charter is our promises to you.

Accessibility
We commit to being accessible.
This means:
Your mentor will be available at the times they have specified to you.
If your mentor can't help you with what you need, they will find someone who can.

Confidentiality
We commit to being trustworthy.
This means:
You can trust us.
We will offer you a confidential space for discussion.
We will protect your personal information.
We will store records securely.
You can have access to your information at any time.
We will not disclose your confidential information unless we are required by law to do so.

Relevance
We will deliver mentoring that is relevant to you.
This means:
We will listen to you.
We will work with you on your goals and priorities.
We will aim to make a difference, as determined by you.

Our mentees also have responsibilities, and they are to:
- Treat your mentoring partnership with care.
- Honour your commitments.
- Let your mentor or the program coordinator know if you opt out of the program before the end of the year.
- Protect your mentor's privacy by not conveying to others any disclosures that could be confidential.

Feedback on our performance
Ensuring quality mentoring is a priority of our program. We welcome feedback so that we can improve the mentoring we provide to you. We will collect and use your feedback to improve how we deliver mentoring. We will review this charter annually.

© State of Queensland (Queensland Health) and Dianne Salvador 2011-2013

Figure 15. The charter of the Doctors for Doctors mentoring program.

The action plan

Table 3 shows the action plan, that is the dimensions of action and corresponding activities that contribute to the Doctors for Doctors mission.

Table 3. The Action Plan of the Doctors for Doctors mentoring program.

Dimension	Activities
Gaining sponsorship	Submit proposal
Recruiting mentors	Advertise for mentors Select mentors Notify applicants of outcome of selection process Issue orientation pack Obtain signed mentor agreements
Training mentors	Design training Organise training logistics Deliver training Evaluate training Establish community of practice Run mentor meetings
Attracting mentees	Promote program Advertise for mentees
Forming partnerships	Matching Introduce mentors and mentees Provide mentees with Charter
Mentoring service delivery	Mentoring conversations
Communicating with mentors	Maintain contact details list Invite mentors to meetings Send meeting minutes Maintain contact with mentors Provide certificate of participation Provide letter of thanks Provide letter of reference
Information management	Obtain secure storage Store personal information securely
Maintaining the program's profile	Purchase and distribute mentor badges Develop and display mentor posters Create a website Send mentees reminders of the program Advertise and host events
Evaluating the program	Form questions Collect data Analyse and interpret data Decide the future of the program: continue as is, adjust and continue, or discontinue Report on findings

The implementation plan

The plan for distributing the workload of the program, mobilising resources, taking action to schedule, and measuring performance and results is the implementation plan, as shown in Table 4.

Table 4. The Implementation Plan of the Doctors for Doctors mentoring program.

IMPLEMENTATION PLAN				
Dimension and activities	Responsibility	Materials	Timeframe	Results measures
Gaining sponsorship: Submit proposal	Coordinator	Email	Term 1	1 x proposal per year
Recruiting mentors: Advertise for mentors Select mentors Notify applicants of outcome of selection process Issue orientation pack Obtain signed mentor agreements	Coordinator	Ads Summary of Duties & Confidentiality Agreement Charter	Term 5, year before	Recruit fifteen mentors
Training mentors: Design training Organise training logistics Deliver training Evaluate training Establish community of practice Run mentor meetings	Coordinator & Educator	Training materials Certificates of Participation Mentor Pre- and Post-Training Questionnaires	Term 1	Group training option Self-paced learning option Administer 1 x survey of mentors before and after training 1 x meeting per term
Attracting mentees: Promote the program Advertise for mentees	Coordinator & Mentors	Ads Mentee EOI forms	Term 1	1 x presentation by coordinator 1 x mentor Q&A forum All interns receive invitation to register
Forming partnerships: Matching Introduce mentors and mentees Provide mentees with charter	Coordinator	Mentor Bio Mentee EOI Charter	Term 1	Matching as per mentee specifications Assign mentors a maximum of five mentees
Mentoring service delivery: Mentoring conversations	Mentors	Record of Encounter Mentoring Delivery Record	Terms 1-5	2 x contact per year, minimum Mentee-centred Aligns with ACFJD Cycle of Caring
Communicating with mentors: Maintain contact details list Invite mentors to meetings Send meeting minutes Maintain contact with mentors Provide certificate of participation Provide letter of thanks Provide letter of reference	Coordinator	Email Phone Recognition of Service Certificate	Terms 1-5	1 x contact per term 1 x meeting minutes per term Issue: • Letter of reference • Letter of thanks • Recognition of Service Certificate

Dimension and activities	Responsibility	Materials	Timeframe	Results measures
Information management: Obtain secure storage Store personal information securely	Coordinator & Mentors	Secure storage	Terms 1-5	As per charter
Maintaining the program's profile: Purchase and distribute mentor badges Develop and display mentor posters Create a website Send mentees reminders of the program Advertise and host events	Coordinator & Mentors	Posters Badges	Terms 1-5	1 x networking event 2 x poster display 5 x newsletter feature Offer all mentors a badge
Evaluating: Form questions Collect data Analyse and interpret data Decide the future of the program: continue as is, adjust and continue, or discontinue Report on findings	Coordinator & Mentors	Mentor Experience Questionnaire Mentee Experience Questionnaire Coordinator's Annual Mentoring Delivery Log Mentor Training Pre-Test and Post-Test Questionnaires	Terms 1-5, monitoring Term 5, end-of-year evaluation	Administer: • 1 x survey of mentors • 1 x survey of mentees Report to mentors and sponsor

Mentor duties

Mentor duties are to:

1. complete mentor training
2. develop mentoring relationships with prevocational doctors with the aim of supporting professional development, career advancement and well-being
3. be available to deliver mentoring at the times they specify
4. contact mentees either individually or as a group, twice or more during the year
5. develop and maintain supportive relationships with fellow mentors
6. communicate with the coordinator during the year
7. participate in program evaluation
8. maintain strict confidentiality about mentees' disclosures as per the Confidentiality Agreement.

Mentor training

Mentors are taught to consider three parallel streams of processes relevant to their mentoring: mentoring service delivery, self-awareness and self-care, and administrative tasks, all examined with reference to the stages of the Cycle of Caring. They choose between participation in a group training session or self-paced learning.

Training content, structured according to the Cycle of Caring, is shown in Table 5.

Table 5. The map of mentor training content for the Doctors for Doctors mentoring program.

Cycle of Caring Stage	Doctors for Doctors Mentor Training Overview		
	Cycle of Caring Approach		
	Mentoring	Self-awareness and self-care	Admin
Empathic Attachment Essence: Open-mindedness Trusting, collaborative alliance A balance between professional under-attachment and over-attachment.	Actions: Building trust Establish an agreement covering initial – goals needs anticipated length of partnership frequency of meetings means of contact boundaries e.g. time, place Assess readiness to change and prepare to work at that level	Actions: Know yourself Manage counter-transference	Actions: Mentoring agreement (optional) Record of encounter (optional) Mentoring delivery record Store records securely
Active Involvement Essence: Continuous attachment Consistent, sustained caring Share a vision and work towards it Support-challenge balance	Actions: Key communication skills – Active listening i.e. attending, following, reflecting e.g. empathy statements Questioning Informing Facilitating brief interventions for goal achievement, learning, insight, clinical reasoning and well-being	Actions: Manage somatic empathy by – un-mirroring arousal awareness sensory anchors strengthening observer dual awareness mindfulness (Rothschild, 2006)	Actions: Assess effectiveness of mentoring encounter Record of encounter (optional) Mentoring delivery record Store records securely
Felt Separation Essence: Let go of active emotional burdens and richness of relationship Separate well Be energised by the professional loss process Be able to reconnect to another and start the cycle again (Skovholt, 2005)	Actions: Conclude mentoring partnership Refer on if required	Actions: Acknowledge feelings Recognise achievements Ending ritual	Actions: Assess effectiveness of mentoring partnership Store records securely

The mentoring

Mentoring takes place from January one year to January the next year, across the junior doctor calendar. Mentoring is available on weekdays or as specified by each mentor.

Mentee-initiated contact frequently relates to career advancement goals. Most contact takes place in the form of 'corridor conversations', that is, opportunistic mentoring.

Defining success

Success for Doctors for Doctors means that:

- All interns are offered suitable support.
- Mentoring partnerships are established as safety nets or active partnerships.
- Mentors are trained in the artful use of conversation, and are ready to respond constructively to the individual needs of mentees.
- Mentors use their example, presence and words.
- Mentoring conversations are helpful to mentees, as determined by the mentees.
- Mentors feel rewarded by the program.
- The program self-sustains, and willing mentees graduate to mentor roles.

The program's ongoing evaluation has shown that Doctors for Doctors has achieved success in all these ways.

Success factors

In Chapter 5 we introduced the fundamentals of mentoring program development, which we discovered through developing Doctors for Doctors. They are:

- Understand your target group and their needs.
- Gain organisational support.
- Appoint a coordinator.
- Have engaged and effective mentors.
- Build the program from a vision.
- Manage risks.
- Treat the program as a year-long renewable project.
- Position the program.

These fundamentals are integral to Doctors for Doctors and its success. Here are some ways in which we apply these fundamentals within Doctors for Doctors.

We know our target group

Interns are our target group. To understand interns, we build relationships with them, have conversations with them, and get to know them. Each term and at the end of the year we seek their feedback about particular aspects of their experience. We also access findings of prominent agencies in relation to junior doctor needs. These actions give us insight into the junior doctor experience.

Executive management provides organisational support

We made an initial proposal to executive management, showing the program's relevance to our organisation's strategic plan. The proposal was successful in gaining the support of executive management. Each year, we confirm the continuation of executive management's support for the program.

The program has a coordinator

We have a designated coordinator with allocated time to devote to the program. The coordinator oversees design and implementation of the program in accordance with the implementation plan. During implementation, the dual focus of the coordinator is managing risk to mitigate the effects of uncertainty on mentoring service delivery, and supporting mentors so they can support mentees.

Mentors are engaged and effective

Mentors are postgraduate year 2 (PGY2) and above, not long out of internship, and they remember what it is like to be an intern. They are selected for their goodwill towards their junior peers and their ability to engage constructively with the program and their mentees. Many have past experience as mentees. They aim to make a difference, as determined by their mentees.

The mentors' effectiveness is enhanced by training that teaches the artful use of conversation. They learn to have transformational conversations with mentees by mixing and matching listening, questioning and informing within the trusting relationship formed by the Cycle of Caring. With just these elements they are able to facilitate outcomes such as goal achievement, learning, insight, clinical reasoning and well-being. The mentors' resilience is enhanced by training in self-awareness and self-care.

The mentors know it can be difficult for interns to ask for help, so they sometimes make the approach and keep it casual.

The program is built from a vision

Our design grew from a vision of resourceful, resilient and effective junior doctors. The design, consisting of the vision, mission, action plan and implementation plan, is cohesive. The vision translates to the mission, which becomes the action plan and is further developed into the implementation plan. The charter is a centrepiece of the design, communicating program commitments, expectations and values to all participants.

We manage risk

Our implementation plan is fortified by a commitment to being aware of and managing risk. Clinical demands are the major source of uncertainty that potentially affect mentoring service delivery. We make room for uncertainty by contingency planning, communicating openly, and infusing all dimensions of implementation with flexibility.

The program is a year-long renewable project

We run key program activities concurrent with term dates. An annual cycle allows us to review and revise the program for continuous improvement each year, and start each year afresh. When we try new ideas we look for the effect, with the results of that trial feeding into decisions and changes. Nothing about the mentoring program is random. There are always reasons behind choices. Those reasons can be about values, our discoveries through trial and error, and our success factors - what brings us closer to our definition of success.

The program has a niche

Within the network of junior doctor support services, we position our program so that it interfaces with other services but does not overlap. Our program's point of difference is access to local knowledge and experience, and support for individual needs in relation to professional development, career advancement and well-being goals. Mentors refer mentees to other services as required.

19. Interviews with Mentors of Junior Doctors

The Doctors for Doctors mentoring program provides the context for many mentoring partnerships to flourish. Within this context, the mentors do the work of the program, having transformational conversations – conversations that guide, inspire and heal.

The ten people we are about to introduce you to are exceptional doctors and inspiring mentors. They make a difference in the lives of junior doctors through their example, their presence and their words. In 2013, we asked them to respond to five questions of their choice about their experiences and perspectives of mentoring doctors.

In this chapter, they share their stories in their own words. The mentors, in the order that they appear, are:

- Dr Harris Eyre
- Dr Joel Wight
- Dr Chris Aubrey
- Dr Jamie-Lea Whyte
- Dr Ching-Siang Cheng
- Dr Sean Chan
- Dr Matthew Oates
- Dr Richard Gartrell
- Dr Rob Mitchell
- Dr Anthony Silva

Dr Harris Eyre
Doctors for Doctors mentoring program
Mentor, 2013

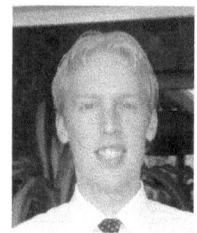

Dr Harris Eyre has broad interests in psychiatry, neuroscience, public health, and medical education. He is currently a Principal House Officer in Psychiatry within the Townsville Health and Hospital Service, Queensland. He is also a PhD Candidate in psychiatric neuroscience at The University of Adelaide, and the Academic Representative for the Townsville Hospital Doctors Society. Dr Eyre has been involved in a variety of medical education-related activities such as clinical and research skills teaching, mentoring, and policy development. He is particularly interested in enhancing doctor well-being, clinical-academic pathways, and portfolio careers in medicine.

What are the most common presenting issues?

"How do I learn the hospital's clinical processes?" To this question I generally suggest politely asking and establishing rapport with the health professionals involved in particular clinical processes. For example, writing prescriptions can be daunting initially; however, the ward pharmacist is always happy to provide advice and support. Interns can also ask their seniors, particularly other junior medical officers. At the end of the day, there's no point floundering with these issues when there are people around who can help out!

"How do I deal with demanding clinical staff (i.e. supervisors, nursing staff, allied health)?" This is a challenging issue, and one that even the most experienced doctors struggle with. It is important for interns to feel supported when dealing with these situations. They must feel free to debrief with mentors or other colleagues. It is important to break down issues and to understand the factors which may have led to this issue, i.e. overworked staff, fatigue, personality factors, lack of mutual understanding of an issue. Through understanding causative factors, interns can begin to deal with these situations in a more appropriate way.

"How do I get onto my desired training program?" Learning how to get onto a program is complex. When interns ask this question I usually offer them my knowledge of the process and suggest they read over the respective college website, then I link them in with a colleague of mine who is already in that program. Alternatively, interns should be empowered to contact the department head or college training representative to discuss this. Basic tenets of getting onto a program include: carrying out courses related to that training program, getting involved in some research, focusing on being a solid clinician in the hospital (as references are key) and getting involved in medical education or other community activities. Of course, an intern must be careful not to 'burn out' in the pursuit of a training program.

What do you see as the advantages of a formal mentoring program over informal mentoring?

There are obviously advantages to both, and both are needed in the hospital; however, formal mentoring programs such as Docs for Docs has a number of key advantages. This allows for pre-determined mentor-mentee relationships whereby the mentor has offered their time and has provided contact details for mentees; the mentee has outlined their interest in mentorship. This suggests there is a will from both parties to engage meaningfully. The Docs for Docs program selects the most appropriate mentors and matches them to related mentees. Finally, the Docs for Docs program offers an avenue to discuss and reflect upon their mentoring experience, as well as guidance on how to improve.

What are some of the ways that a mentoring program can improve the experience of junior doctor?

Mentoring programs assist interns by providing an avenue for pastoral and professional support. In my experience, mentoring helps lower intern stress levels, outlines and explains the complex world of hospitals and medicine, and links interns into a larger social network within the hospital.

What type of person makes the best junior doctor mentor?

There is no 'best' junior doctor mentor as all mentors can provide unique perspectives and supports based on their past experiences and interests. However, some core attributes include willingness to mentor, approachability, warmth, developed empathic listening skills, and the ability to provide measured advice without overstepping one's knowledge/experience level. Another key skill is to be able to link interns in to other experts in the field.

What motivates most to become mentors?

There are multiple reasons for most people becoming a mentor. The most important driver is wanting to provide a supportive and safe learning and working environment for juniors. All mentors have been through the 'fires' of the internship, and we all know how tough it can be - support and guidance are key. Therefore, why not give to those currently going through those trials? Of course, this concept of helping those more junior to us is ingrained into the medical profession's ethos - we innately do it because it's right. Mentoring and knowing you've made a positive contribution to someone's career gives you a sense of purpose and satisfaction. Another common reason for becoming a mentor is the inclusion of the activity on one's CV.

Dr Joel Wight
Doctors for Doctors mentoring program
Mentor, 2012 and 2013

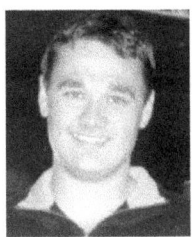

Occupation: Haematology Advanced Trainee
Age: 28
Graduated: James Cook University 2008
Years mentoring: 3
I enjoy: Church, snowboarding, and date nights with my wife.
Why am I a mentor? Being a junior doctor is tough. It can feel very lonely. It's great to help people through.

What are some of the ways that a mentoring program can improve the experience of junior doctor?

Mentoring programs provide a real safety net for junior doctors. As a junior doctor, encountering potentially serious things that you've never had any experience with is a daily occurrence. This is a struggle that most people are unwilling to admit to their peers. It's kind of like sitting in a lecture theatre where the lecturer is banging on about some nonsense that nobody understands, but nobody is willing to ask in front of the crowd because they think they're the only one who hasn't gotten it. Having someone more experienced to debrief with about these experiences is helpful not only for educational reasons; it does wonderful things for your mental health.

What are some of the things you tell your mentees that you wish someone told you?

Medicine is a tough career, and feeling completely out of your depth is homogenous. You need to come to terms with this early and realise that you're going to feel this way for about the next 10 years (or longer!)

The two most important qualities in medicine are honesty and humility. You need to be honest with yourself about your own limitations, honest with your patients, honest when you don't know what's going on, and honest when you have made a mistake. You will learn much faster when you're honest! And no matter how amazing you become, you must remain humble. Arrogance is the enemy of quality practice. A surgeon who believes himself too skillful to have a complication will not recognise a complication when it comes. A physician who believes himself to have made the correct diagnosis will not consider new evidence that suggests otherwise. There is no place in medicine for arrogant doctors – so don't become one.

Just because your consultant says it, doesn't make it true. Consultants are fallible human beings just like the rest of us.

What are your top three tips for mentee self-care?

1. Most of the time when your colleagues get angry, it's because they are busy and stressed and out of their depth. Just like you are. Try to remain civil with one another.
2. Get some good rest and have an interest outside of your work. It will make you a better doctor and a happier person.
3. Ask for help before it all becomes too much. People don't fall in a heap all at once – it's usually a build-up of things. Kids on bikes get the "speed wobbles" before they actually fall off. It's much better to correct the speed wobble than to have to get back on the bike cut, bruised and bleeding.

What type of person makes the best junior doctor mentor?

Approachable, with some free time. Someone willing to share their own personal experience. Someone real – honest and humble. A role model in life and in work. Usually such a person struggled through being a junior doctor themselves and has learned the hard lessons!

Do you use written agreements with mentees? Why/why not?

Personally, I don't. I think a written agreement tends to defeat the purpose of the mentoring relationship. It makes the process too formal. We're not counsellors, we're mentors. A formal mentoring program is a great idea for the reasons of structure, support and access. However, the mentoring relationship fails fundamentally if the mentee feels as though they can't approach the mentor on a personal level. It isn't easy but we have to resist the bureaucrats and lawyers.

Dr Chris Aubrey
Doctors for Doctors mentoring program
Mentor, 2011

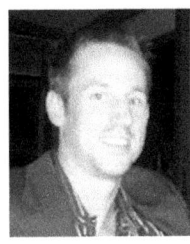

Chris graduated from James Cook University in 2008 and commenced his training at the Townsville Hospital where he influenced a number of improvements for junior doctors in his role as the Doctors Society president. In 2011 he was accepted onto the General Surgery Program and moved to Brisbane to commence his training. Despite his love for surgery, the long hours impacted on Chris's lifestyle, prompting him to make the big decision to pull out of the training program. Chris now lives in Brisbane, working as a surgical assistant, which gives him the luxury of enjoying a healthy work-life balance.

How do you think a mentoring program is beneficial?

Often junior doctors can lack insight into what career opportunities exist, what these opportunities are really like, and how they can gain access into these careers. With working in the hospitals for a few years comes knowledge of some of these specialties. A mentoring program bridges this gap and can also provide further introductions to help facilitate a smoother career path.

What advice would you offer junior doctors to get the most out of mentoring?

Take advantage of talking to others that have more experience than you - even if only by a year or two. Every year after graduation has its own unique challenges, and the quickest way to learn these challenges is talking to those who have experienced them.

What are the most common issues you have addressed as a junior doctor mentor?

1. Discussed decisions about which career path to choose.
2. Overcoming personality clashes with other staff members.
3. Opportunities for research or other methods of boosting a CV.

Where is your most common meeting place for mentoring encounters?

In a hospital common room, cafe, ward halls. Not all encounters need to be formal, or even confidential, so being adaptable and sensitive to the needs of the mentee is key.

What are the top three challenges faced by junior doctors?

1. Deciding which training program they want to enter.
2. Finding out exactly what needs to be done to be accepted onto the program.
3. Putting in the hard work to get accepted, while keeping up with everyday demands of the job.

Dr Jamie-Lea Whyte
Doctors for Doctors mentoring program
Mentor, 2012

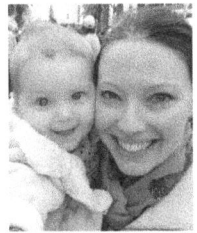

Jamie-Lea Whyte is a GP registrar who undertook her internship and most of PGY2 at the Townsville Hospital. She studied medicine at Griffith on the Gold Coast. She has returned to the local neighbourhood, working at the Gold Coast Hospital fulfilling the rest of her prescribed hospital time before entering into GP land to pursue the rest of her training. She is a huge advocate for GP training and was The Townsville Hospital's GP Ambassador for 2012 – an initiative of GPRA (General Practitioner's Registrar's Australia) and the Going Places Network. This program is aimed at being a link within hospitals to the infamous and mysterious land of General Practice training. As is evident, Jamie is a big believer in work-life balance that she recognised is quite hard to come by in hospital career pathways, even when you've reached the top. When not doing ward call on weekends, she's relaxing on a beach basking in the sun with her family, dreaming about part-time training ahead...

What are some of the things you tell your mentees that you wish someone told you?

Intern year and residency is really about determining which career path of training you would pursue in medicine. It's not so much about what rotations you *liked* to do, but also paying attention to what rotations you *didn't like*. I found that the best feedback about these decisions was simply by asking my spouse/family – "During which rotations was I a better person to live with?" If they were hiding from me when I arrived home after working a surgical shift...then I took that as a sign for my future career options...! Work-life balance is the key! - Your family/partner knows you best!

Why did you sign up to being part of the formal mentoring program?

I found this opportunity a great way to connect with other interns who are about to/are walking the path I had just trod. The issues I faced through intern year were vivid and easily accessed to assist others in transitioning from student life to full-time work (and responsibilities). It was my way of giving back – proof that you can survive intern year and that it does get easier.

What are the top three challenges faced by junior doctors?

1. Ever-changing routines (rotations changing every ten weeks) – this impacts on home life and work-life balance (and your body clock). I personally felt like intern year was like having five different jobs.
2. Time poor – at work when you're there, and at home (*if* you're there!)
3. Adjusting and coping with hospital life! The politics at times is frustrating and battling the many egos…(including my own I'm sure!)

What is a typical day in the life of a junior doctor?

Coffee on board, arriving on time, preferably early. Being organised and on top of the patients' situations from the night before. Having a load of blank forms ready to go prior to ward round. Go from there – the day usually declares itself!

Why do you think some junior doctors don't seek help when they need it?

I believe there is no understanding of what 'help' means. Is it an ear to listen or someone to actually solve a problem? Most times of feeling like we need 'help' are probably to do with a personal side of the job (such as: I am not coping with this amount of stress, or, I am feeling frustrated that my expectations of my role are not what is the actual case). These personal issues are often difficult to own because you are often wondering if you should just carry on because it's only a 'job'. We are our own worst enemy whereby seeking help is almost like admitting defeat. Just as plumbers usually have the leakiest taps, so doctors tend to have the poorest of health. This is a reflection of our reluctance to seek help, be it for physical, emotional, or psychological well-being. Unfortunately, this attitude does not promote longevity in our careers and only encourages burnout…

Dr Ching-Siang Cheng
Doctors for Doctors mentoring program
Mentor, 2012

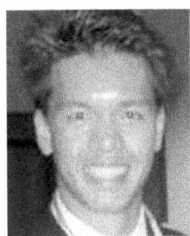

University: The University Of Queensland School Of Medicine, graduating class of 2009

Current Hospital: The Royal Perth Hospital (2013)

Current Specialty: General Surgery Registrar SET 1 in 2013; accepted into Vascular Surgery SET 2 in 2014

Current interests: Family time, reading surgical textbooks, learning languages, and also racing multi-sport events if not on-call.

What are the most common presenting issues?

People approach mentors for different reasons. Most of the people who approached me were former international students like myself and who were likewise keen on getting into surgical training. I was also approached by local graduates (i.e. Australians) who were keen on getting into surgical training. As a successful applicant I offered advice on how to get involved in research, publishing, and which courses one should attend, just to name a few. None of what I can give is unique, but it is aimed to provide the prospective candidates (and colleagues) a reference point.

How do you think a mentoring program is beneficial?

It allows for an informal exchange of information and follow-up of those mentored. As the doctors functioning as mentors are marginally more senior than those mentored, it also gives them a more recent perspective of "what is to be done."

Who was a mentor to you and what did they help you with that you remember the most?

I have benefited from mentorship from consultants who I have remained close friends with – it is absolutely crucial to have someone you can speak to outside your training field, but who is a surgeon, who can give you another perspective of what is needed to be done. I had a few mentors: A Cardiothoracic surgeon, a Gynecologist, a Vascular surgeon and a Colorectal surgeon. I was also close friends with a Vascular Fellow and another Cardiothoracic Registrar. They were important in moulding my decision to enter surgical training – and I regularly update and seek their opinion on various issues in general – be it surgical conduct and training, issues in the workplace, ideas for presentations, and even just for a casual chat.

What does the ideal mentoring service for junior doctors offer?

I think that the team approach would work best. A mentoring team should be assembled to consist of members with various strengths and interests – to give as wide a spectrum of choices to the junior doctors as possible.

Why did you decide to get involved as a mentor in the Doctors for Doctors mentoring program?

There is a substantial population of former international students from Australian medical schools who head to The Townsville Hospital for their internship. It is a great location for training and for getting onto competitive programs nationally. Former international students face additional challenges in getting onto programs, or sometimes even settling into a regional Australian community – most of them have not lived outside of major Australian cities!

As an involved member (Club Medical Officer & Patrol Lifeguard) of the Townsville Surf Lifesaving Club and an active participant in local running and swimming events, I felt that I could give encouragement to former international students to step out and become involved in the wider community beyond medicine. It also helps them fit into the community. As an aside, sporting achievements and community service also contribute to the scoring of the curriculum vitae in some surgical specialty applications…

Dr Sean Chan
Doctors for Doctors mentoring program
Mentor, 2013

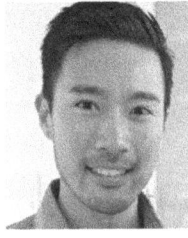

Dr. Sean Chan graduated from the University of Queensland in 2011 and has since lived and worked in North Queensland. He is currently a Junior House Officer at the Townsville General Hospital and has aspirations to become a clinical urologist. He is actively involved in teaching, research, and community work for the Prostate Cancer Foundation of Australia and as a volunteer firefighter for the Rural Fire Service of Queensland. He comes from a diverse background and has spent much of his life in Singapore, Canada and Australia.

What are the most common presenting issues?

Junior doctors are extremely varied and come from different educational and social backgrounds. Career guidance and work-life balance questions have probably come up the most but a lot of the people that access the mentorship program are also new to the city or Australia in general. I commonly get asked for advice on suburbs to live and places to eat.

Who was a mentor to you and what did they help you with that you remember the most?

As I am interested in urology, I was happy to find out that my mentor was a PHO in Surgery. I had a lot of ideas about what I thought was important for getting onto a surgical program, but it was my mentor who sat me down and told me what was and was not important, what I should focus on, and where to start. The thing I remember the most was him being accepted onto the general surgical program. Before he left, he gave me many of his surgical textbooks, and at that point I felt that with the books and his advice I had all the tools necessary to succeed.

What are some of the ways that a mentoring program can improve the experience of junior doctor?

The program offers support and guidance during a significant transitional period from student to doctor. Having a mentor allows junior doctors to access professional advice from doctors who have recently progressed through this time. The program allows you to have a point of contact who is not intimidating and is in touch with current practice of junior doctors.

What advice would you offer junior doctors to get the most out of mentoring?

I think it's important to have a clear idea about issues that are important to you and to schedule in regular catch-up times for discussion. Setting up regular meetings with flexible times and locations is also desirable to cater for conflicting schedules.

Why do you recommend junior doctors access mentoring?

New medical school graduates face many new responsibilities, experiences and challenges, which can be overwhelming. Mentees can take advantage of the experience of other doctors who have faced these same challenges in their career and feel a sense of support and belonging to their profession.

Dr Matthew Oates
Doctors for Doctors mentoring program
Mentor, 2013

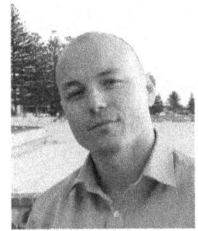

Dr Matthew Oates is from the surfing town of Kangaroo Island in South Australia. After high school Matthew delayed further studies to surf, travel overseas and teach English in Honduras, Central America. On returning to Australia he studied Bachelor of Medical Science at Flinders University in Adelaide, before settling on medicine as his chosen career. He completed the MBBS program at Griffith University on the Gold Coast in 2011 and moved to Townsville for intern year at The Townsville Hospital in 2012. Matthew's belief in the importance of doctors supporting each other and having a positive attitude towards healthcare motivates him to mentor junior doctors and medical students. Matthew currently works as a Junior House Officer at The Townsville Hospital and is pursuing training in cardiothoracic surgery.

Do you enjoy being a mentor? If so, why?

I enjoy being a mentor because...

Being a mentor creates an opportunity for the mentee to evaluate things from a different perspective, to think about past events that the mentor may have personally experienced or seen others experience. Revisiting these thoughts and hearing feedback from a different point of view can be refreshing.

By listening to mentees about the experiences that they have gone through and how these things have affected them, how they have felt at times, how they have endured or overcome events, whether with humour or determination, can be inspiring. At times the conversation can shed light on similar experiences that I have had, allowing for personal development for the mentee, and potentially skills to approach similar trials in the future differently.

Mentoring is not solely conversations about the work environment. Mentoring incorporates other aspects of what a career is, a lifestyle. Everyone in a demanding career is juggling social environment, study, relationships and personal time along with work. Positives to discussing medicine and life surrounding the pursuit of medicine, reveals the motivation that brought both of you to your career in the first place.

By listening and discussing these things with someone there is a strong level of shared honesty. I believe for my own health as well as the mentee's health, that whatever the conversation reveals there is a responsibility to find a positive aspect to these experiences. If the experience is a good one, then the responsibility is to validate the achievement of the person as an individual and to bolster their motivation and confidence to achieve even more. If their experience is negative, then it's to frame the experience for them to give them the realisation that even the worst of experiences and conundrums can be overcome. Or if there is an ongoing struggle, then it's to reveal similar experiences that you have had to them, to assure them that they are not alone in what they are going through and that other people struggle with similar difficulties. By approaching interactions with mentees in such a way a number of things happen. There is a strength in giving strength to others, and there is a unification for yourself as well as others in recognising that your peers are remarkable people who are extremely resilient.

Our career is emotionally and physical demanding and these interactions allow people to discuss how the job and aspects of life are affecting them, and in ways vent things in an accepting, safe environment.

What are your top three tips for being an effective mentor?

1. Listen

    Know when to listen and know when to talk. It may seem simple but can often be difficult to do. Allow the person you are speaking with to express themselves. Work on making them feel heard and understood. It's your role.

2. Have good judgement but don't judge.

    Approach your mentee openly and allow them to express themselves in an environment they feel safe in. Put any personal negative internal responses that may come up aside and stay focused on the goal. Help them to grow positively. It's their right.

3. Educate

   Enable mentees to learn, whether academically or in other ways, with links to resources. Discuss tools that help you cope or learn. Give tips on healthy eating, exercise or outlets that help you to function in an optimal way both physically and mentally.

   To effectively communicate, it is essential that your mentee feels safe. Remember that these interactions reveal a vulnerability that requires confidentiality, something that you should be familiar with as a health worker.

What are the skills you draw on most as a mentor?

Life experience and transparency are more approaches than skills. Keeping these things in the back of your mind helps with communication and flow of conversation.

Why did you decide to get involved as a mentor in the Doctors for Doctors mentoring program?

The transition from student to doctor was not an easy one for me and in retrospect I would have benefited from having a mentor. I believe that the experiences that I have had are not dissimilar to the experiences that many other people on the same path undergo. This industry benefits from healthy healthcare workers and at times the job can be personally isolating. I wanted to support the people around me so that negative experiences that they had could be discussed to reduce negative impacts on their lives.

Dr Richard Gartrell
Doctors for Doctors mentoring program
Mentor, 2012 and 2013

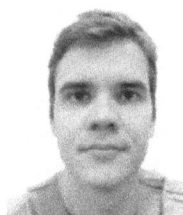

I am originally from Brisbane but studied at Griffith on the Gold Coast. I moved to Townsville for my internship for a variety of reasons but predominately because it was a busy tertiary hospital that would provide a variety of new experiences and challenges in my early career. My PGY2 year offered me the opportunities I needed to pursue general surgery and the exposure and training that I have received in Townsville has facilitated the transition to a PHO role for 2013.

What are the most common presenting issues?

The common theme for mentees was predominantly regarding prospective career paths. Given the increased competition for training places, the majority of junior doctors were looking to the future and eager to place themselves in a favorable position for subsequent employment. I found that being in a similar position and learning from my own experiences, I was hopefully able to offer them topical advice.

How well-prepared do you feel as a mentor to respond to junior doctor needs?

I feel the ability to help junior doctors comes predominantly through prior experience and a degree of approachability. A substantial proportion of our knowledge comes from learning from mistakes and therefore the experience of others. I felt I could relate to their concerns, given I had experienced the same issues as a junior doctor. Therefore, the issues that were raised did not come as a surprise. Approachability is perhaps more innate and pertains to a level of trust and how you are perceived by colleagues. Should the mentees have your trust, the relationship becomes far more constructive.

What are your top three tips for mentee self-care?

1. Maintain an open mind, i.e. try to get as much broad exposure as possible without becoming fixated on a single career path. People's attitudes change over time, and you may be surprised.
2. Have as many interests outside of the hospital as possible. Try to avoid talking shop with colleagues when in a social environment.
3. Immerse yourself in all opportunities inside the hospital, and look after your physical health outside of it. Best achieved with a group of friends – not necessarily medically trained.

Do you use written agreements with mentees? Why/why not?

No. My approach was mostly informal and hopefully more relaxed. I think written agreements would deter mentees from further approaches given the perceived pressure associated with written agreements.

Where is your most common meeting place for mentoring encounters?

Any place that serves coffee.

Dr Rob Mitchell
Mentor, 2011, 2012 and 2013

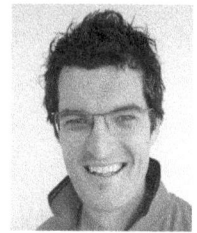

Rob Mitchell is an Emergency Registrar at The Townsville Hospital and Immediate Past Chair of the AMA Federal Council of Doctors in Training. He has been involved in medical education and professional representation activities since medical school, during which he served as President of the Australian Medical Students' Association.

Rob continues to work with national bodies involved in health professional education and workforce, and sits on committees of the Department of Health and Ageing and the Australian Medical Council. Outside of his representative responsibilities, Rob has assisted in the coordination of teaching programs at Monash University and is a founding partner of Cor Mentes Health Consulting. He also serves as a Director of the Global Ideas Forum, an event that aspires to link early career professionals with opportunities in international health and development.

What are the best things about being part of a mentoring program as a mentor?

I see mentoring relationships as mutually enhancing, rather than unidirectional. I'm an informal mentor to several medical students and junior doctors, and I often worry that I get more out of the relationship than they do!

Mentoring is not a role that I have actively sought, but I have found it thoroughly rewarding. There is something inspiring about hearing the plans and aspirations of recent graduates. It also encourages you to reflect on your own ambitions and career goals.

In various situations, the mentees I'm affiliated with have provided me with guidance and advice. This has often been in relation to advocacy issues and representation of junior doctors, when it's often helpful to have another perspective. In one case, we have worked together to produce policy documents and articles, and our different experiences have enhanced the quality of the product.

Most of the mentoring arrangements I have been a part of have quickly evolved into friendships, which reflects the reciprocal nature of the relationships. This won't be appropriate in all circumstances, but as a trainee myself, it has been a natural progression.

Who was a mentor to you and what did they help you with that you remember the most?

On several occasions, I have identified a need for mentoring and an appropriate mentor, but have been reluctant to approach them for advice and support. I regret this, as the value in mature mentoring relationships can be immense. If I could have my time again, I would have the confidence to approach the potential mentor and ask them for guidance.

Despite my unwillingness to self-initiate formal mentoring relationships, there are several individuals who I identify as mentors. These are mainly doctors who I have worked with, in both clinical and non-clinical capacities, and respect immensely. It's become apparent that they all share certain qualities: they are humble, hard-working and approachable, and maintain the highest of professional standards. They are typically involved in public health pursuits, are passionate about education, and have a vision for the future.

I have gained a great deal from working with these individuals, and their informal guidance has been invaluable in negotiating professional challenges and making important decisions. The value of role-modelling cannot be underestimated.

Everyone's ideal mentor is different: the attributes I have described above may not be attractive to other trainees. I would encourage all junior doctors to identify potential mentors, and whether as part of a formal mentoring relationship or not, utilise their experience and expertise. Doctors are remarkably willing to give of their time for trainees and medical students.

How do you stay engaged with your mentees?

Each mentor and mentee relationship will function differently. I think it's important that arrangements develop organically and reflect the requirements of both parties.

I've found that informal arrangements generally work well, with one party contacting the other at important junctures. My mentee catch-ups are generally over coffee – but that may just reflect a penchant for caffeine!

Regular communication is important, but emails and phone calls don't have to be long or detailed. Everyone who I have nominally mentored has been involved in interesting pursuits and initiatives – so there is always something to talk about, and a great incentive to catch up!

Would you describe your mentoring style as active or passive?

It's probably evident from the comments above that my style is generally passive. This reflects a view that a mentor's responsibility is to meet the needs of the mentee and not the other way around.

The dynamics in every mentoring arrangement will be different, but I think there is value in allowing the relationship to evolve naturally. I think there are risks with being too rigid, and forcing engagement can be counterproductive. There is nothing worse than a stiff conversation that neither party wants to participate in!

By the same token, mentoring partnerships, like all relationships, need care and commitment – so it's important to make sure that contact is relatively regular. Even a simple SMS (or email, Facebook message or tweet!) can be sufficient to touch base and ensure that the mentee is in a good place.

What drew you to becoming a mentor?

It was never a conscious decision. I was still at university when a more junior medical student asked if I would be their mentor. We had many mutual interests and lots to offer one another in terms of sharing knowledge and experience.

Despite that, I failed to deliver by neglecting to maintain regular contact. I didn't place sufficient priority on the relationship, and it petered out as a result. All mentoring partnerships will have a natural history – some will endure, others will diminish – but this one ended prematurely. I was too focused on my own activities, and failed to appreciate the value in learning from someone else.

This was a helpful experience in that it has (hopefully) improved my performance as a mentor. As my own career progresses, the value of mentoring is becoming more apparent – which has inspired me to maintain regular contact with medical students and junior doctors, both in a mentoring capacity and otherwise.

We can all learn a lot from each other's experiences. In my mind, mentoring relationships provide immense benefits for both the mentor and mentee, including opportunities to reflect, inspire, and collaborate. Is there a downside?!

Dr Anthony Silva
Doctors for Doctors mentoring program
Mentor-elect, 2014

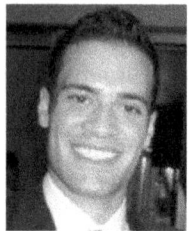

Education: MBBS – The University of Queensland (2012), MSc – Queen's University (2010)

Current Hospital & Position: The Townsville Hospital; Intern

Career Aspirations: Orthopaedic Surgery

Previous Mentorship Experience:

International Peer Advisor – The University of Queensland, School of Medicine (2010-2012). Mentored future and current international medical students at The University of Queensland.

Peer Mentor Team Leader – The Hotel Dieu Hospital Student Auxiliary (2008-2009). Designed, implemented, and participated in a large Peer Mentorship program providing advice, guidance, and support for student volunteers working at the hospital.

Why did you decide to get involved as a mentor in the Doctors for Doctors mentoring program?

A career in medicine can be quite challenging at times. Intern year is certainly no exception and marks a great transition point from being a medical student to taking on the full responsibilities of being a doctor and caring for patients as part of a team. It is easy to understand how this transition could be quite challenging for some new graduates and how without a strong support network or appropriate guidance, that the workload and pressures of the new job could become overwhelming.

I decided to become involved in the program so that I could share my experiences with the new junior doctors starting their medical careers, and provide them with the support and guidance that can help them achieve a successful and enjoyable year.

What do you see as the advantages of a formal mentoring program over informal mentoring?

While I believe informal mentoring is very important, and partake in the practice as both a mentor and a mentee myself, formal mentorship programs fill a very important void in the support networks for junior doctors.

Formal mentorship programs bring together people looking for guidance and support and those willing to share their time and experiences. I believe this is most important for those junior doctors who may not feel comfortable reaching up the medical hierarchy to seek advice or support in situations where their peers may not have the experience to give appropriate guidance.

Additionally, in having a mentor arranged through a formal program, a support network is already in place for this group of junior doctors; allowing them a comfortable medium to access support which they may otherwise perceive as inaccessible.

What are the biggest challenges of being a mentor in a formal mentoring program?

I believe the biggest challenge in a formal mentorship program arises from the nature of the program itself. While an informal mentoring relationship develops naturally between likeminded or compatible individuals, a formal mentorship program may pair two people with different personalities or viewpoints. These situations can be quite challenging for a mentor. In situations where this dichotomy exists in a mentoring relationship, I've found that although the relationship can be more challenging initially, in being mindful and dedicating more energy into understanding the dichotomy of views, that these challenging relationships can become quite successful.

Do you use written agreements with mentees? Why/why not?

I do not use written agreements with my mentees. I prefer to discuss with my mentees what they would like to get out of the mentor-mentee relationship and verbally agree on the frequency and nature of meetings. I view written agreements as placing a businesslike burden on the relationship, making meetings more of a chore, rather than the supportive and hopefully enjoyable process that it can be.

How well prepared do you feel as a mentor to respond to junior doctor needs?

Every mentee's needs are different, so it can be hard to feel totally prepared to meet their needs. Drawing on my own experiences as a junior doctor, the guidance and support I've received, my previous experience as a mentor, and the training from the Doctors for Doctors program I feel that only the experience itself could prepare me more.

Epilogue

Imagine a teaching hospital where the sharing of knowledge and expertise is the cultural norm and readily given, where collaboration rather than competition is the driving force of progress, where conversations are constructive and lead to learning, insight and effective action, where a culture of care permeates the work environment, and patients do well as a result. How good would that be?

This is not just wishful thinking; it is a real possibility for the future, and a mentoring program at your teaching hospital can contribute to making the vision a reality.

We have guided you along the path which we have taken to develop a successful junior doctor mentoring program, so that you can too.

You now know how to design a program by formulating a vision, mission and action and implementation plans. You may have completed your program design using the design worksheets and templates we provided in Appendix 2, being the *Vision, Mission and Charter worksheet*, the *Charter template*, the *Action Plan template* and the *Implementation Plan template*. If you would like more inspiration, consider the design ideas from the Doctors for Doctors mentoring program featured in Chapter 18.

You also know how to proceed with the implementation phase and manage the program as a strategy, a network, a context and an investment.

We have offered you our ideas and experience, and we have featured interviews with mentors of junior doctors. Now it is time for you to take action. From here, let your implementation plan be your guide.

We wish you success.

Appendices

Appendix 1 – Coordinator's Checklist

Mentoring program design

- ✓ Vision
- ✓ Mission and charter
- ✓ Action plan
- ✓ Implementation plan
- ✓ Re-vision after the first round of implementation

Sponsorship

- ✓ Proposal

Recruitment of mentors

- ✓ Send out an EOI request to prospective mentors
- ✓ Select mentors
- ✓ Notify mentor applicants of the outcome of their application
- ✓ Issue orientation pack
- ✓ Obtain signed mentor agreements

Attracting mentees

- ✓ Advertise the program to mentees

Forming partnerships

- ✓ Matching
- ✓ Introduce mentors and mentees
- ✓ Provide mentees with charter

Training

- ✓ Seek executive management's approval to release mentors for training
- ✓ Send invitation to training
- ✓ Design training

- ✓ Deliver training
- ✓ Evaluate training
- ✓ Issue a starter kit
- ✓ Establish community of practice
- ✓ Run mentor meetings

Communicating with mentors

- ✓ Ask for information
- ✓ Give information
- ✓ Issue invitations
- ✓ Issue reminders
- ✓ Give appreciation

Information management

- ✓ Storage system for records

Maintaining the program's profile

- ✓ Purchase and distribute mentor badges
- ✓ Produce and display posters
- ✓ Create a website
- ✓ Send mentees reminders of the program
- ✓ Advertise and host events

Evaluating the program

- ✓ Form questions
- ✓ Collect data
- ✓ Analyse and interpret data
- ✓ Share findings
- ✓ Make a decision about the future of the program: continue as is, adjust and continue, or discontinue
- ✓ Produce report

Appendix 2 – Worksheets and Templates

Chapter 6 – The 4-Step Design Process
Vision, Mission & Charter worksheet — 180
Action Plan template — 181
Implementation Plan template — 182
Charter template — 183

Chapter 8 – Gaining Sponsorship
Proposal template for start-up/first year — 184
Sample proposal for continuation of the program — 185

Chapter 9 – Recruiting Mentors
Mentor Bio form — 186
Summary of Duties and Confidentiality Agreement — 187
Sample First Meeting Plan — 188

Chapter 10 – Attracting Mentees
Expression of Interest – Mentee — 189

Chapter 11 – Forming Partnerships
Matching worksheet — 190
Partnerships summary — 191

Chapter 12 – Training 'Ready for Anything' Mentors
Training Calendar — 192
Sample Training Run Sheet — 193
Mentor Pre-training Questionnaire — 194
Mentor Post-training Questionnaire — 195
Certificate of Participation — 196
Community of Practice Sample Meeting Plan — 197

Chapter 13 – Mentoring Service Delivery
Mentoring Agreement template — 198
Record of Encounter — 199
Mentoring Delivery Record — 200

Chapter 14 – Communicating with Mentors
Recognition of Service Certificate — 201

Chapter 17 – Evaluating the Program
Mentor Experience Questionnaire — 202
Mentee Experience Questionnaire — 203
Coordinator's Annual Mentoring Delivery Log — 204
Annual Report template — 205

CHAPTER 6

Vision, Mission and Charter Worksheet

Your vision

Describe what your junior doctor community wants to become.

Your mission

Describe how your program will make the vision a reality, in terms of what you will deliver, how you will deliver it, and who you will serve.

What –

How –

Who –

Your extended mission – your charter

Now develop your mission further into commitments to mentees who access the service. Take your top three (or more) values and write them as commitments.

Value:

We commit to (describe what you will do):

This means (now be really specific about what you will do):

(Repeat for as many commitments as you'd like to make.)

Action Plan Template

Dimension	Activities
Gaining sponsorship	
Recruiting mentors	
Training mentors	
Attracting mentees	
Forming partnerships	
Mentoring service delivery	
Communicating with mentors	
Information management	
Maintaining the program's profile	
Evaluating the program	

CHAPTER 6

Implementation Plan Template				
Dimension and activities	Responsibility	Materials	Timeframe	Results measures
Gaining sponsorship:				
Recruiting mentors:				
Training mentors:				
Attracting mentees:				
Forming partnerships:				
Mentoring service delivery:				
Communicating with mentors:				
Information management:				
Maintaining the program's profile:				
Evaluating the program:				

CHAPTER 6

Charter Template

[Mentoring program] Charter

We are committed to providing junior doctors with [type of support]. Our Charter is our promises to you.

[Value]

We commit to...

This means:

[Value]

We commit to...

This means:

[Value]

We commit to...

This means:

Our mentees also have responsibilities and are to:

Feedback on our performance

Ensuring quality mentoring is a priority of our program. We welcome feedback so that we can improve the service we provide to you. We will review this charter annually.

CHAPTER 8

Proposal Template for Start-Up/First Year
[Hospital, Mentoring Program, Year]

Contents

Program overview

- What you are proposing (the strategy/potential solution)
- Why you are proposing it (the need, the impacts of the need, the evidence for the solution and the alignment with other strategies)

Approach, phases, timelines

- How you will take action
- When you will take action

Staffing and management plan

- Who will take action

Resources: costs and returns on investment

- How much it will cost
- How it will be beneficial
- How you will measure the effects

Managing risks

- Risks
- How you will manage risks

© State of Queensland (Queensland Health) 2011-2013

CHAPTER 8

Sample Proposal for Continuation of the Program

Dear [Executive],

I am seeking your approval for the continuation of [Unit's] popular [Mentoring program] in [Year]. In our [number of years] year of offering the program, the demand has been remarkable with [percentage of] Interns seeking a mentor through the program in [Year]. In this email I will include some details of the program and the benefits and the costs for your consideration.

Program overview

[Mentoring program] is a mentoring program based at [Hospital]. The program offers junior doctors a blended professional development and employee well-being service, provided by their senior colleagues. The program:

- harnesses the capabilities of volunteer mentors
- embeds the mentoring service within a robust system of support and training for mentors
- is underpinned by a sustainable model of service delivery; mentees become mentors
- is designed, delivered and evaluated by one unit [Unit] with clear lines of responsibility and accountability
- actions the recommendations of key junior doctor well-being literature.

Benefits

The potential benefits of the program are numerous and include improvements in the emotional health of prevocational doctors, patient safety, performance and productivity, morale and job satisfaction, attractiveness of [Hospital] as an employer, workforce retention and cost savings.

[Work unit] is continuing to collect program evaluation data to ascertain the effects of [Mentoring program] on mentees and [Hospital]. Our key performance indicators to date have been the number of volunteer mentors, mentoring partnerships, mentoring encounters, and mentees becoming mentors. Together these show significant uptake of mentoring services and support for the program.

Costs

The costs of the program relate to:
Staffing – Mentor and mentee time participating in mentoring encounters: [approx. hours] hours per term; coordinator time: [approx. hours] hours per week.
Training – Venue hire and catering for mentor training: [amount] dollars. The training event is followed by one meeting of [minutes] duration per term.
Incidentals –– Stationery and mentor badges: [amount] dollars.

Could you please confirm your support for the continuation of the program in [Year]?

Kind regards,

[Coordinator]

© State of Queensland (Queensland Health) 2011-2013

CHAPTER 9

Mentoring is a partnership between a mentor and a mentee that creates a space for conversation and a potential for development of the mentee.

Mentees can approach their mentor to discuss issues, explore ideas, ask for feedback, set and pursue goals, and voice their experiences.

Mentors are available to listen, provide constructive feedback, and facilitate development according to the needs of mentees.

Please use this form to provide some information about yourself that can be used for program advertising and facilitating contact by mentees.

Mentor Bio

Name:

PGY2/3+ (please circle)

My Alma Mater (where I went to Med School):

About me (hint: a short blurb – 50 words or less, e.g. "Since graduating from James Cook University, Townsville I have developed a real passion for junior doctor education and well-being as well as women's health. I plan to apply for the obstetrics and gynaecology program in the near future. Any questions or need help, come and have a chat.")

Preferred contact details (hint: can be via switch):

Times available:
and or
Times unavailable:

Terms I've completed:

My career goals:

Special interests/things I can help mentees with:

[Mentoring program]

© State of Queensland (Queensland Health) 2011-2013

Summary of Duties

1. Complete mentor training
2. Develop mentoring relationships with prevocational doctors with the aim of supporting professional development, career advancement and well-being, according to the charter
3. Be available to deliver mentoring at the times you specify
4. Contact your mentees, either individually or as a group, a minimum of twice per year
5. Develop and maintain supportive relationships with fellow mentors
6. Communicate with the coordinator during the year
7. Participate in program evaluation
8. Maintain strict confidentiality about mentees' disclosures as per the following Confidentiality Agreement

Confidentiality Agreement

[Mentoring program] protects the confidentiality of all mentees and mentors.

Mentors are required to acknowledge and agree to the following:

- I will not discuss any information concerning my mentees with anyone outside [Mentoring program]. If I need to talk about mentees within [Mentoring program], I will not reveal identifying information.
- I understand that I am required to disclose confidential information regarding a mentee in the following circumstances:
    i. where there is a serious risk that a mentee will be of harm to themselves or others
    ii. where a mentee has made a written request for information to be released
    iii. where a mentee discloses notifiable conduct
    iv. a court has ordered that information be released or disclosed.
- I understand that any breach of confidentiality (except as stated above) constitutes grounds for termination of my involvement with [Mentoring program].

I agree to the statements contained within the [Mentoring program] Confidentiality Agreement.

Date: _____

Name (please print): _____ Signature_____

Please provide a signed copy of this form to [Coordinator], [Mentoring program], [Hospital].

© State of Queensland (Queensland Health) 2011-2013

Sample First Meeting Plan

Goals

- Get to know each other
- Identify the why, what, who, how of our mentoring program
- Plan Mentor training

Ice-breaker activity – Think of a secret

1. Think of a secret you have never told anyone/something you would find it difficult to talk about. *You will not be asked to reveal this at any time in this exercise.*
2. Look around the group and think about which person in the group you would tell your secret to if you had to tell one person. *Do not reveal who this person is.*
3. Now think about what it is about that person that made you choose him or her.
4. Call out attributes of the person you have chosen.
5. Give the list a title e.g. The Qualities of a Mentor
6. Debriefing. Draw attention to this: all the qualities we need are in this room, and together we can learn skills to create and deliver something important.

Answer these questions

- **Why** have this program? e.g. Develop effective, resilient, resourceful doctors. Discuss.
- **What?** Activity: "If I were a mentee." Picture yourself as a mentee. Think of some problems you have had to grapple with or are struggling with right now. Jot down words, phrases, or simple sentences. What would I want to get out of seeing a mentor? Scope of program, limits to service, what mentoring is, what it isn't? Discuss.
- **Who?** Who would you like to assist? Target group and needs? Discuss.
- **How?** How would I want to be treated? How would you like to assist? What training will enable you to deliver on mission? In what format? Discuss.

© State of Queensland (Queensland Health) 2011-2013

CHAPTER 10

Mentoring is a partnership between a mentor and a mentee that creates a space for conversation and a potential for development of the mentee.

Did you know...
[Hospital] has a mentoring program – [Mentoring program]

Mentees can approach their mentor to discuss issues, explore ideas, ask for feedback, set and pursue goals, and voice their experiences.

Mentors are available to listen, provide constructive feedback, and facilitate development according to the needs of mentees.

Use this form to register your interest in becoming a mentee. The [Mentoring program] Coordinator will match you with a mentor and provide you with details for initiating contact. Alternatively, you may nominate your preferred mentor.

Expression of Interest – Mentee

Name:

My Alma Mater (where I went to Med School):

I am seeking a mentor who is (please indicate):

- Male
- Female
- Either male or female
- PGY2
- PGY3+
- Either PGY2 or PGY3+
- any specialty
- _____ specialty

and who is available:

- Once per month
- Once per term
- Occasionally/on an irregular basis
- In person
- By phone
- By email

Preferred mentor name (if known):

My email address is:

My phone number is:

[Mentoring program]

© State of Queensland (Queensland Health) 2011-2013

CHAPTER 11

Matching Worksheet

Profile (year, specialty)	Mentor Name	Mentee-Mentor Partnership	Mentee Name	Specifications (gender, year, specialty)

CHAPTER 11

Partnerships Summary	
Mentor **& contact details**	**Mentee** **& contact details**

WORKSHEETS AND TEMPLATES

CHAPTER 12

Training Calendar

Term	Event	Topic/s	Venue
1	First meeting		
1	Mentor training		
2	Term 2 meeting		
3	Term 3 meeting		
4	Term 4 meeting		
5	Term 5 meeting		

Sample Training Run Sheet

	[Mentoring Program] Training [Date]
Time	**Topic**
12.30pm	Arrivals, lunch
1.00pm	Welcome Introduction: how to serve as a mentor to doctors, format of session
1.10pm	Share an understanding of mentoring Reflect on experiences of receiving mentoring Identify principles of effective mentoring Meet Dr X (case)
1.30pm	Communication and relational work in mentoring
2.00pm	The Cycle of Caring and Empathic Attachment
2.15pm	Active Involvement and the work of mentoring: facilitation
2.45pm	Mental health first aid
3.00pm	Felt Separation and concluding the partnership
3.15pm	Afternoon tea
3.30pm	Self-awareness and self-care
3.55pm	Admin
4.00pm	Theory into practice: mentor Dr X
4.15pm	Looking back, looking forward
4.25pm	Evaluation
4.30pm	Close

CHAPTER 12

Mentor Pre-training Questionnaire

1. What does the term mentoring mean to you?

2. How confident are you to provide mentoring?

    ☐ not confident
    ☐ somewhat confident
    ☐ confident
    ☐ highly confident

© State of Queensland (Queensland Health) 2011-2013

Mentor Post-training Questionnaire

1. What does the term mentoring mean to you?

2. What did you learn at the mentor training day on [date]?
    - ☐ Mentoring knowledge and skills
    - ☐ Communication knowledge and skills
    - ☐ Facilitation knowledge and skills
    - ☐ Self-awareness knowledge and skills
    - ☐ Self-care knowledge and skills
    - ☐ Other (please specify):

3. How confident are you to provide mentoring now?
    - ☐ not confident
    - ☐ somewhat confident
    - ☐ confident
    - ☐ highly confident

4. Was the training adequate preparation for commencing mentoring?   Yes   No

5. Was the training accessible?   Yes   No

6. Was the training length suitable?   Yes   No

7. Do you have any suggestions for changes to the training for future programs?
    If so, list them here:

Thank you for your feedback.

© State of Queensland (Queensland Health) 2011-2013

Certificate of Participation

This is to certify that

Dr [Mentor]

has successfully completed

[Mentoring program]
Mentor training

at [Venue]
on [Date]

having attended [number] hours of training
and completed all group work

- The Cycle of Caring approach to mentoring
- Communication and facilitation skills
- Self-awareness and self-care
- Admin skills

_____   _____
[Coordinator]   [Director of Clinical Training]

© State of Queensland (Queensland Health) 2011-2013

CHAPTER 12

Community of Practice Sample Meeting Plan

Welcome, catch-up.
Topic of the Day/activity. Topic of the Day is your choice/mentor's choice/sample Topic of the Day if no one has ideas.
Close.

Sample Topic of the Day is "Powerful Questions."

Intro (as a visual display on a whiteboard):

Mentoring is a vehicle for insight and action.
Relationship is a key success factor for mentoring (vertical arrow down to...)
Communication a key relationship success factor (vertical arrow down to...)
Listening and questioning the key communication success factors for mentoring (which brings us to...)
Powerful questions.

A famous example of why powerful questions matter: Watson & Crick asked, "What might DNA look like in 3D form?" leading to the discovery of the double helix.

Reflection question: Think of a mentoring experience, formal or informal, that went well (went well = led to a breakthrough insight or action, transformation). What question catalysed this result? (Share reflections.)

Brainstorm: What makes a question powerful for catalysing insight and action?

A powerful question:
- Is thought-provoking
- Channels attention and focuses enquiry
- Generates curiosity
- Surfaces underlying assumptions
- Invites creativity and new possibilities
- Generates energy and forward movement
- Evokes more questions

Sample questions* for breakthrough insights or actions during future mentoring encounters –

Questions for insight:
"What is it we're not seeing?"
"What's emerging here for you?"
"What's been your/our major learning, insight, or discovery so far?"
"What else do we need to think about?"

Questions for action:
"What's possible here and who cares?"
"What needs our immediate attention going forward?"
"What unique contribution can we each make?"
"What conversation, if begun today, could ripple out in a way that would create new possibilities for the future of (your situation)?"

Consider other applications/areas of work or personal life where powerful questions for insight and action could come in handy. (Share ideas.)

*Questions taken from *The Art of powerful questions* (2003), a World Café publication by E. Vogt, J. Brown and D. Isaacs, retrieved from www.theworldcafe.com

CHAPTER 13

Mentoring Agreement Template

Between _____ & _____

Purpose of mentoring: (please indicate)

___ professional development

___ career advancement

___ well-being

Goals (if known):

Mentor commitments:

Mentee commitments:

Method/s, frequency, and available times of communication:

Duration of mentoring:

Signed: [Mentor]   [Mentee]

Date:

© State of Queensland (Queensland Health) 2011-2013

CHAPTER 13

Record of Encounter

Mentee Code:

Date:
Time:
Duration of encounter (minutes):

Mentee:
Gender: M / F
Post-graduate Year: 1 / 2 / 3
Session: First / Follow-up
Discussion topics (please circle):

Work
Protocols and procedures
Relationship – peer
Relationship – supervisor
Culture
Career
Med Admin
Performance
Stress
Other_____

Personal
Friendships
Family
Health
Mental health
Parenting
Drug and alcohol
Finances
Other_____

Type of encounter (please circle):
Face-to-face meeting
Phone
Email
Other_____

Notes:

© State of Queensland (Queensland Health) 2011-2013

CHAPTER 13

Mentoring Delivery Record [Mentor]					
Communication method	**Minutes**				
	Term 1	Term 2	Term 3	Term 4	Term 5
Face-to-face					
Email					
Phone					
Other					
Topics	**Frequency**				
	Term 1	Term 2	Term 3	Term 4	Term 5
Work Protocols and procedures Relationship – peer Relationship – supervisor Culture Career Med Admin Performance Stress Other					
Personal Friendships Relationships – family Health Mental health Parenting Drug and alcohol Finances Other					
No. of mentees:					

Instructions for mentors:
During the year, make an entry on this record for each mentoring encounter.
First, **record the duration of the encounter in minutes**, using the field that applies to the term and the communication method.
Then, **tally the topic/s of conversation** discussed during the encounter.
Record in the bottom row the number of mentees who accessed mentoring during the year.

CHAPTER 14

Recognition of Service Certificate

[Hospital]

[Mentoring program]

[Hospital] would like to formally acknowledge and thank

Dr [Mentor]

for [his/her] participation in, and dedication to, [Mentoring program] in [year]

_____   _____

[Coordinator]   [Executive/Sponsor]

[Hospital logo]

© State of Queensland (Queensland Health) 2011-2013

CHAPTER 17

Mentor Experience Questionnaire

Mentoring delivery

Was your mentoring role rewarding? (please circle)   Yes / No

What was most rewarding about being a mentor in the program?

Please comment on the suitability of your mentoring partnerships

Approximately how many hours of mentoring did you deliver this year?

Overall, how would you rate the mentoring program for mentees? (please circle)
                    Inadequate / adequate / more than adequate

Would you volunteer to serve as a mentor again? Why or why not?

Please list any suggestions for future programs:

Mentor training and support

Was the initial training adequate to prepare you for mentoring? (please circle)   Yes / No

Did the community of practice meetings each term assist you to continue your mentoring? (please circle)   Yes / No

Were the meetings each term accessible? (please circle)   Yes / No

Overall, did you receive the support you needed to be a mentor? (please circle)   Yes / No

Please list any suggestions for training and support for future programs:

Thank you for your feedback.

© State of Queensland (Queensland Health) 2011-2013

CHAPTER 17

Mentee Experience Questionnaire

About you: (please circle)
    Male / female
    PGY: 1 / 2 / 3
    IMG: Yes / No

About your mentoring experience:

How many mentoring encounters did you have?: (please circle)   1 / 2-5 / 6-10 / 10+

Was your mentoring partnership suitable? (please circle)   Yes / No
Comments:

In general, did your mentor listen to you and respond constructively? (please circle)
Yes / No

Was your mentor available when you needed them? (please circle)   Yes / No

Did you and your mentor discuss topics important to you? (please circle)   Yes / No

Did mentoring contribute to positive changes in your life this year? (please circle)
Yes / No
Comments:

Did mentoring help you to transition from medical school to the workforce?
(please circle)   Yes / No
Comments:

Do you have any concerns about your mentoring experience or the program in general? (please circle)   Yes / No
Comments:

After your mentoring experience, would you considering becoming a mentor in the program? (please circle)   Yes / No

Please list any suggestions for future programs:

Thank you for your feedback.

© State of Queensland (Queensland Health) 2011-2013

CHAPTER 17

Coordinator's Annual Mentoring Delivery Log

Mentor	Minutes per term					
	T1	T2	T3	T4	T5	Total
M1						
M2						
M3						
M4						
M5						
M6						
M7						
M8						
M9						
M10						
Total						

Topics	Frequency per term, all mentors					
	T1	T2	T3	T4	T5	Total
Work Protocols and procedures Relationship – peer Relationship – supervisor Culture Career Med Admin Performance Stress Other						
Personal Friendships Relationships – family Health Mental health Parenting Drug and alcohol Finances Other						
Total no. of mentees						

Instructions for the coordinator:
Use this form in conjunction with the completed Mentoring Delivery Records.
First, record the **mentoring delivery in minutes**, using the field that applies to the term and the mentor.
Then, record the tally of the **topic/s of conversation** for all mentors.
Record in the bottom row the total number of mentees who accessed mentoring during the year.

Annual Report Template

[Year] program overview

Purpose of the evaluation

Evaluation results

   Process evaluation

- Questions and answers re: inputs/activities/outputs –

- Contextual factors –

   Outcome evaluation

- Questions and answers re: effects –

Interpretation of findings

- Our definition of success for the program is –

- We achieved success in –

- Limitations of the evaluation -

Recommendations

We recommend continuing/changing/discontinuing –

Glossary

3 Cs	The coordinator's main tasks for the design and implementation phases of a mentoring program: communicating, connecting and communicating some more.
4-step design process	Vision formulation, mission formulation, action planning and implementation planning.
Action plan	The list of dimensions of action and corresponding activities that will contribute to the delivery of the mission.
Action planning	Developing the mission into an action plan, by listing the dimensions of action and corresponding activities that will contribute to the delivery of the mission.
Activities	In a process evaluation, activities are processes that generate the program's services and products.
Charter	The program's set of commitments to mentees.
Coordinator	The representative of the organisation who takes overall responsibility for the design and implementation of the mentoring program.
Implementation plan	A plan for distributing the workload of the program, mobilising resources, taking action to schedule, and measuring performance and results.
Implementation planning	Expanding the action plan into an implementation plan, by identifying the plan for distributing the workload of the program, mobilising resources, taking action to schedule, and measuring performance and results.
Informal mentoring	Mentoring that takes place organically without the involvement of a coordinator.
Inputs	In a process evaluation, inputs are the financial, material and human resources invested in the program.
Junior doctor	A doctor undertaking prevocational medical training.
Junior doctor year	One year apportioned into five terms, usually spanning from January in one year to January in the next year.

Mentee	The less experienced professional in the mentoring partnership.
Mentor	The more experienced professional in the mentoring partnership; in a junior doctor mentoring program the mentor is a doctor with general registration (more than one year experience) who is interested in helping junior doctors at the start of their career.
Mentoring	A trusting partnership between a more senior professional (mentor) and a less senior professional (mentee), and a developmental process for the benefit of the mentee.
Mentoring encounter	A mentor's contact with a mentee that relates to mentoring.
Mentoring program	A strategy, a network of relationships, a context and an investment designed to facilitate mentoring; directly, through assistance with beginning, maintaining and concluding partnerships, and indirectly, through sponsorship, communication, promotion, information management, and evaluation.
Mentoring program development	A process of mentoring program design and implementation, producing a mentoring program.
Mentoring Program Development Model	A representation of the design and implementation phases of a mentoring program for junior doctors.
Mentors' mentor	A senior doctor who agrees to act as a support person to mentors.
Mission	The work that will make the vision a reality.
Mission formulation	Translating the vision to a mission by describing what the program does, how it does it, and who it does it for.
Orientation pack	A package for new mentors containing program information and agreements for signing including an agreement to perform mentor duties, to maintain confidentiality and to uphold the charter.
Outcome evaluation	An evaluation process that explores effects: whether the mentoring had an effect on participants and brought about the intended changes.
Outcomes	In an outcome evaluation, outcomes are the effects of program outputs.
Outcome indicators	Outcomes indicators are the specific, observable measures of outcomes used in an outcome evaluation.
Outputs	In a process evaluation, outputs are services and products that the program provides.

Process evaluation	An evaluation process that explores whether the mentoring implementation took place as planned, and the extent to which it reached its target group of junior doctors.
Process indicators	Process indicators are the specific, observable measures of inputs, activities and outputs used in a process evaluation.
Re-vision	A suitable design for the next year of the program.
Re-visioning	Re-visioning is a design review process in preparation for the next year of the program.
Sponsor	A representative of the organisation who has the authority to approve funding of programs.
Starter kit	A set of post-training mentoring resources that can consolidate mentors' learning and further guide them as they begin to establish mentoring partnerships.
Sponsor	A representative of the organisation who has the authority to approve funding of programs.
Target group	A group of people sharing a common characteristic or set of characteristics, that the program seeks to reach.
Values	Values are the ideals that underpin the program and the ideals of behavior that the coordinator and the mentors agree to enact.
Vision	A vision for a community is an image of what that community wants to become.
Vision formulation	Identifying an image of what a community wants to become.

References

Australian Medical Association. (2013). *2012 AMA Junior Doctor Training, Education and Supervision Survey: report of findings, March 2013*. Retrieved from https://ama.com.au/2012-ama-junior-doctor-training-education-and-supervision-survey

Australian Medical Association. (2011). *Health and wellbeing of doctors and medical students, 2011: AMA position statement*. Retrieved from https://ama.com.au/position-statement/health-and-wellbeing-doctors-and-medical-students-2011

Australian Medical Association. (2008). *AMA survey report on junior doctor health and wellbeing*. Retrieved from https://ama.com.au/ama-survey-report-junior-doctor-health-and-wellbeing

Australian Public Health Nutrition Academic Collaboration. (2005). *A mentoring framework for public health nutrition workforce development.* Retrieved from http://www.inclentrust.org/uploadedbyfck/file/compile%20resourse/new-resourse-dr_-vishal/Mentoring%20framework%20for%20nutrition.pdf

Berg, K. & Latin, R. (2007). *Essentials of research methods in health, physical education, exercise science and recreation* (3rd ed). Sydney: Lippincott, Williams & Wilkins.

beyondblue (2013). *National Mental Health Survey of Doctors and Medical Students, October 2013.* Retrieved from http://www.beyondblue.org.au/docs/default-source/default-document-library/bl1132-report---nmhdmss-full-report_web.pdf?sfvrsn=2

Centers for Disease Control and Prevention. (2008). *Introduction to process evaluation in tobacco use prevention and control, February 2008*. Retrieved from U.S. Department of Health and Human Services website: http://www.cdc.gov/tobacco/tobacco_control_programs/surveillance_evaluation/process_evaluation/pdfs/tobaccousemanual_updated04182008.pdf

Confederation of Postgraduate Medical Education Councils. (2006). *Australian Curriculum Framework for Junior Doctors*. Fitzroy: CPMEC.

Doherty, C. (2004). Introducing mentoring to doctors. *Development and Learning in Organizations, 18*(1), 6-8.

Gawande, A. (2007). *Better: A surgeon's notes on performance.* New York: Metropolitan.

Harris, R. (2007). *The happiness trap.* Wollombi: Exisle Publishing.

Hayes, S. & Smith, S. (2005). *Get out of your mind and into your life: The new acceptance and commitment therapy.* Oakland CA.: New Harbinger Publications.

International Organization for Standardization and Standards Australia International. (2009). *Risk management: Principles and guidelines* (ISO 31000: 2009). Geneva: ISO.

Kirkpatrick, D. L. (1967). Evaluation of training. In R. Craig & I. Mittel (Eds.), *Training and development handbook* (pp. 87–112). New York: McGraw Hill.

Kumar, R. (2010). *Research methodology: A step by step guide for beginners* (3rd ed.). Los Angeles: Sage.

Lake, F.R. & Ryan, G. (2004). Teaching on the run tips 3: Planning a teaching episode. *Medical Journal of Australia, 180,* 643-644.

Levinson, D. J. (1978). *The seasons of a man's life.* New York: Knopf.

MacDonald, G., Starr, G., Schooley, M., Yee, S.L., Klimowski, K., & Turner, K. (2001). *Introduction to program evaluation for comprehensive tobacco control programs.* Atlanta, GA: Centers for Disease Control and Prevention.

MacLeod, S. (2007). The challenge of providing mentorship in primary care. *Postgraduate Medical Journal, 83,* 317-319.

National Health and Medical Research Council. (2014). *Ethical considerations in quality assurance and evaluation activities, March 2014.* Retrieved from http://www.nhmrc.gov.au/_files_nhmrc/publications/attachments/e111_ethical_considerations_in_quality_assurance_140326.pdf

Neher, J.O., Gordon, K.C., Meyer, B., & Stevens, N. (1992). A five-step microskills model of clinical teaching. *Journal of the American Board of Family Practice, 5*, 419-24.

Office of the Information Commissioner Queensland. (2012). *What is personal information?* Retrieved 28 April 2014, from http://www.oic.qld.gov.au/guidelines/for-community-members/Information-sheets-privacy-principles/what-is-personal-information

Rothschild, B. (2006). *Help for the helper*. New York: W.W. Norton & Company.

Sambunjak, D., Straus, S.E., & Marusic, A. (2006). Mentoring in academic medicine: A systematic review, *Journal of the American Medical Association, 296* (9), 1103-1115.

Schön, D. A. (1987). *Educating the reflective practitioner*. San Francisco, CA: Jossey-Bass.

Skovholt, T.M. (2005). The cycle of caring: A model of expertise in the helping professions. *Journal of Mental Health Counseling, 27*, 82-93.

Triola, M. & Triola, M. (2013). *Biostatistics for biological and health sciences with Statdisk* (Pearson New International ed.). Sydney: Pearson.

Vogt, E., Brown, J. & Isaacs, D. (2003). *The art of powerful questions: Catalyzing insight, innovation, and action.* Retrieved from World Café: http://www.theworldcafe.com

Webb, P. & Bain, C. (2011). *Essential epidemiology: An introduction for students and health professionals* (2nd ed.). Cambridge: Cambridge University Press.

Whitmore, J. (2009). *Coaching for performance*. London: Nicholas Brealey Publishing.

Index

This is an index to subjects. Only significant cited works and their authors have been indexed. A full list of citations is provided in the *References* section. Figures are indicated by the letter 'f'. Tables are indicated by the letter 't'.

A

about the authors 223
abstract actions in mentoring 83f
Acceptance and Commitment Therapy 86t
accessibility (charter) 137f
ACFJD see Australian Curriculum Framework for Junior Doctors (ACFJD)
acknowledgements xiii
Action plan template 181
action planning, defined 207
action plans 42, 44f, 49, 53
    defined 207
    Doctors for Doctors mentoring program 138t
active involvement (Cycle of Caring) 85, 87, 95, 141t
activities, defined 207
AMA see Australian Medical Association (AMA)
2012 AMA junior doctor training, education, and supervision survey 11–12, 20
AMA survey report on junior doctor health and wellbeing 14, 22
Annual report template 130, 205
APHRA see Australian Health Practitioner Regulation Agency (APHRA)
appendices 175–205
assessment processes in hospitals 20, 21
attracting mentees 73–5, 177
    action plan 138t
    implementation plan 139t–40t
    worksheets and templates 189
Aubrey, Chris (mentor), interview 153–4
Australian Curriculum Framework for Junior Doctors 18, 95–6
Australian Health Practitioner Regulation Agency (APHRA) 111
Australian Medical Association (AMA) xvii, 7–8, 17
    2008 survey 7
    2012 survey 11–12
    support for junior doctors 45f
authors, biographical information 223

B

benefits of mentoring 17–24
beyondblue (Beyond Blue Limited) xvii, 7–10, 15, 17, 45f
    2013 survey 9
business case for mentoring programs 66–7

C

career advancement and job security xvi, 10–11, 18, 21, 27, 50, 140
case for mentoring 17–24
    mentoring solution 17–21
    possible results 21–4
Centers for Disease Control and Prevention 117, 120, 123
Certificate of participation (template) 105, 196

Chan, Sean (mentor), interview 159–60
charter 52, 63, 80, 96, 109, 136, 137f, 144
   defined 207
   worksheets and templates 180, 183
Charter template 183
checklist, coordinator's 177–8
Cheng, Ching-Siang (mentor), interview 157–8
clinical reasoning 86t, 144
Coordinator's annual mentoring delivery log (template) 127, 204
Collings, Rachel xi–xii, 10, 11, 12, 22, 223
communicating with mentors 99–106, 178
   action plan 138t
   conversations 127–8
   implementation plan 139t–40t
   information sharing 101–3
   invitations and reminders 103–4
   methods 100
   reasons for 99–100
   schedules 106
   showing appreciation to 105, 201
   worksheets and templates 201
communication channels (email) 70–1, 99–106
community caring role of doctors 6
community of practice 91–2, 102, 106, 138t, 139t
Community of practice sample meeting plan 197
Confederation of Postgraduate Medical Education Councils (CPMEC) 18, 95
confidentiality agreements 72, 109, 139t, 140, 187
confidentiality (charter) 137f
control groups in experimental design 121, 122
conversations with mentors 127–8
coordinator
   checklist for 177–8
   defined 207
   role of xvii, 59–64, 143
coordinator's role, 3 Cs communication tools 60–1

coping strategies for doctors 14–15
CPMEC *see* Confederation of Postgraduate Medical Education Councils (CPMEC)
Cycle of Caring 36–7, 83, 85, 87, 95, 97, 141t, 144
   see also Skovholt, Thomas

D

data analysis and interpretation 128–30
data collection 125–8
DCT *see* Director of Clinical Training (DCT)
dealing with patients 3–4, 4, 5, 6, 10, 13, 24
design review process *see* re-visioning
developmental goals for junior doctors 27, 123
DHAS *see* Doctors Health Advisory Service (DHAS)
Director of Clinical Training (DCT) 135
disclosing information 110–12
doctors, coping strategies 14–15
Doctors for Doctors charter 137f
Doctors for Doctors mentoring program xvi 135–45
   action plan 138t
   annual cycle 144
   charter 136, 137f
   history 135–6
   implementation plan 139–40t
   major focus 135
   mentor training 141t
   program positioning 145
   success factors 142–5
   vision and mission 136
Doctors Health Advisory Service (DHAS) 45f
doctors' home life 10
duties of mentors 72, 139t, 140, 187
duty of care 110–11
duty prioritisation skills 5

E

EDMS *see* Executive Director of Medical Services (EDMS)
email communications 70–1, 101–5
emails, examples of 70, 71, 79, 89, 94, 95,

97, 101–5
emergency medicine 6, 13
empathic attachment (Cycle of Caring) 85, 87, 95, 141t
employee assistance programs, support for junior doctors 45f
end-of-year data collection 126
epilogue 173
ethical considerations of mentoring programs 119
Ethical considerations in quality assurance and evaluation activities 119
evaluating mentoring programs 117–31, 178
    action plan 138t
    continuous improvement 131
    data analysis and interpretation 128–30
    data collection 125–8
    description of 117
    implementation plan 139t–40t
    Mentoring Program Development Model 118–19
    process and outcome evaluation 119–23
    question formation 123–5
    reporting on findings 130–1
    worksheets and templates 202–5
evaluation planning 118f
Executive Director of Medical Services (EDMS) 135
executive management support 40–1, 143
experimental design 121–2, 128
Expression of interest - Mentee (template) 189
Eyre, Harris (mentor), interview 148–50

F

feedback for junior doctors 12, 20, 21
feedback for program (charter) 63, 99, 137f
felt separation (Cycle of Caring) 85, 87, 95, 97, 141t
female doctors, mental health 9
figures and tables 8, 40, 42, 44, 45, 49, 64, 80, 83, 118, 123, 131, 137, 138, 139–40, 141
foreword v-vii

formal assessments for junior doctors 12
forming partnerships 77–81, 177
    action plan 138t
    for and against matching 77
    implementation plan 139t–40t
    introductions 79–80
    matching criteria 77–8
    matching system 78–9
    re-matching 81
    timing for introductions 80
    worksheets and templates 190–1
4-step design process xvii, 49–55
    action planning 53
    defined 207
    implementation planning 53–4
    mission formulation 50–2
    re-visioning 54–5
    vision formulation 50
    worksheets and templates 180–3
fundamentals of mentoring program development 39–45
    annual cycle 43, 44f
    coordinator appointment 41, 143
    engaged, effective mentors 41, 143–4
    gaining organisational support 40–1, 143
    program positioning 44–5, 145
    risk management 43–4, 144
    success factors 142–5
    understanding target group 39–40
    vision 42, 144

G

gaining sponsorship, worksheets and templates 184–5
Gartrell, Richard (mentor), interview 164–5
General Clinical Education Committee (GCEC) 135
general practitioners (GP) 6, 14
    support for junior doctors 45f
glossary 207–9
goal achievement 86t
GROW (goal achievement) 86t

H

Health and wellbeing of doctors and medical students - 2011 7, 14
home life of doctors 10
hospital-based mentoring programs, support for junior doctors 45f
Human Research Ethics Committee (HREC) 118, 119

I

IETP *see* Intern Education and Training Program (IETP)
illustrations list x
impacts of medical practice 7–9
implementation plan 121
 data analysis 128
 defined 207
 example of 139t–40t
 guidelines xvii-xviii
Implementation plan template 182
implementation planning, defined 207
Indigenous doctors, mental health 9
informal mentoring, defined 207
information management 107–12, 177
 action plan 138t
 collecting, using and storing 109–10
 disclosing information 110–12
 implementation plan 139t–40t
 personal information 107–9, 186–9
inputs, defined 207
integration of mentoring and other strategies 40f
Intern Education and Training Program (IETP) 136
international medical graduates 9, 136
internationally trained doctors, mental health 9
interns as mentees 135-136, 143
interpretation of evaluation data 128–30
interviews with mentors of junior doctors 147–72
introduction xv-xix

J

job satisfaction 6, 23
job security and career advancement 10–11, 21
Journal of the American Medical Association (journal article) 22
junior doctor experience xv, 3–16, 143
 career development 135
 challenges of practice 9–14
 coping strategies 14–15
 dealing with patients 4, 5
 impacts of practice 7–9
 rewards of practice 6
 roles 5–6, 13
 support services 15–16, 45f, 145
 survey 7–8
 workloads 13
junior doctor mentoring programs, introduction to xv
junior doctor year 43, 44f, 88, 106
 defined 208
junior doctors
 a day in the life of 3–4
 defined 207
 developmental goals 27, 123
 feedback 20
 formal assessments 12
 interviews with 147–72
 mental health 7–9
 role of 5–6, 13
 skills and processes 18

K

Kirkpatrick Model (evaluation) 125

L

learning activities 89–90
legal advice recommendations 107, 109
lifelong learning 7, 11–12
list of illustrations x

M

maintaining program's profile 113–15, 178
    action plan 138t
    implementation plan 139t–40t
    methods 114–15
matching 77–81, 136
    advantages and disadvantages 77
    criteria for 77–8
    introductory emails 79
    system 78–9
    worksheet 78, 190
Matching worksheet 190
medical practice
    challenges of 9–14
    impacts of 7–9
    rewards of 6–7
mental health in junior doctors 7–10
mentee EOI form 78, 189
Mentee experience questionnaire (template) 127, 203
mentees
    communicating with 74–5
    defined 208
    eligible candidates 136
    exclusion criteria 73–4
    preparing for mentoring 75
    roles and responsibilities 28, 137f
Mentor bio (template) 78, 186
Mentor experience questionnaire (template) 126, 202
Mentor post-training questionnaire 195
Mentor pre-training questionnaire 194
mentor training content 141t
mentoring
    benefits of 17–24
    defined 208
    monitoring and concluding 96–7
    motives for 69
    roles and responsibilities 28
    standards 95–6
Mentoring agreement template 198
Mentoring delivery record (template) 96, 127, 200

mentoring partnerships 25–31
    basic concepts 26–8
    developmental goals for junior doctors 27
    hiking scenario 25
    hospital-based scenario 29–30
    key features 26–7
    schools comparison 34, 59
    support roles 33
mentoring program
    advantages of a formal program 35
    agreements to cooperate 36
    benefits 15
    challenges 37–8
    defined 208
    description of 33–4
    design 177
    ethical considerations 119
    evaluation 117–31
    how it works 36–7
    major focus 135
    promoting 113–15
    questions about xviii
    values 51–2
mentoring program development
    coordinator appointment 41
    defined 208
    engaged, effective mentors 41
    fundamentals 39–45, 142–5
    organisational support 40–1
    risk management 43–4, 144
    understanding target group 39–40
    vision development 42
Mentoring Program Development Model xv-xviii, 42, 54, 131f
    defined 208
    design and implementation phases 42f, 49f
    evaluation 118–19
    figures 42, 44, 49, 64
    five-term junior doctor year 44f
    implementation dimensions 64f
    re-visioning 131f
    risk management 43–4

mentoring service delivery 93–7, 141
    action plan 138t
    encouraging delivery and uptake 94–5
    implementation plan 139t–40t
    monitoring and concluding partnerships 96–7
    services 93–4
    standards 95–6
    worksheets and templates 198–200
    written agreements 198
mentors
    acknowledgment 105, 201
    after initial recruitment 72
    attracting applicants 70–1
    competencies 87
    data collection role 126
    defined 208
    duties and confidentiality agreements 72, 187
    effectiveness of 143–4
    interviews with 147–72
    professional development 84
    reasons for participation xvi
    roles and responsibilities 28, 140
    selection criteria 69, 136
    support for 62, 135
    training of 83–92, 135, 138t, 139t–40t, 141t
    well-prepared 84
mentors' mentor, defined 14–15, 208
minefield game (learning activity) 89–90
mission 42, 44, 49, 50–4
    defined 208
    examples of 136, 138
    worksheets and templates 180
mission formulation, defined 208
Mitchell, Rob (mentor), interview 166–9
monitoring and concluding mentoring 96–7

N

National Health and Medical Research Council (NHMRC) 119
National mental health survey of doctors and medical students 8–10

NHMRC *see* National Health and Medical Research Council (NHMRC)
notifiable conduct 20, 52, 87, 96, 110, 111, 187

O

Oates, Matthew (mentor), interview 161–3
One Minute Preceptor (clinical reasoning) 86t
organisational skills 19
organisational support for mentoring programs 65–7, 143, 177
orientation pack, defined 208
orientation week 80f, 136
outcome evaluation 119–23
    defined 208
    examples of questions 124
    research design 121–2
outcomes, defined 208
outcome indicators 122
    defined 208
outputs, defined 209
overseas trained doctors 9, 136

P

participation, certificate of 105, 196
partnerships, formation 77–81
Partnerships summary (template) 191
patient care 3–4, 5, 6, 10, 13, 24
    well-being 4
personal information 107–9, 186–9
    definition of 107
PGMEU *see* Postgraduate Medical Education Unit (PGMEU)
postgraduate medical councils, support for junior doctors 45f
Postgraduate Medical Education Unit (PGMEU) 135–6
preface xi-xii
process evaluation 119–23
    defined 209
    questions 124t
process indicators 120–1
    defined 209
process and outcome evaluations 123f

examples of questions 124t
professional development 7, 11–12, 84, 145
    community of practice 91–2
program design 47–55
program evaluation 117–31
program implementation 57–131
program profile maintenance 113–15
Proposal template for start-up/First year 184
psychological distress in doctors 7–10, 8f

Q

question formulation (evaluation) 123–5
questionnaires 90, 126–7, 140t, 194, 195, 202, 203

R

Rachel says (quotations) 10, 11, 12, 22
Rachel's story xi-xii
re-vision 42
    defined 209
re-visioning 54–5, 117, 130, 131f
    defined 209
'ready for anything' mentors 83–92, 192–7
Recognition of service certificate (template) 201
Record of encounter (worksheet) 96, 127, 199
recruiting mentors 69–72, 177
    action plan 138t
    email communications 70–1
    implementation plan 139t–40t
    motives and selection criteria 69
    worksheets and templates 186–8
reference list 211–13
reflection-on-action 86t
relevance (charter) 137f
reporting on findings (of program evaluation) 130–1
research design for outcome evaluation 121–2
rewards of medical practice 6–7
risk management 43–4, 62–3, 144
role of coordinators xvii, 59–64
role of junior doctors 5–6, 13

S

Salvador, Dianne 223
Sample first meeting plan 188
Sample proposal for continuation of the program 185
Sample training run sheet 193
scenarios 3–4, 25, 29–30, 34
schools comparisons 34, 59
Silva, Anthony (mentor), interview 170–2
Skovholt, Thomas v-vii, 36–7, 83, 95, 141t
    see also Cycle of Caring
sponsor 65
    defined 209
    reporting to 130
sponsorship 65–7, 113–14, 177
    action plan 138t
    implementation plan 139t–40t
    worksheets and templates 184–5
standards for mentoring 95–6
starter kit 91, 139t
    defined 209
statistical applications for data analysis 128
STOP (Acceptance and Commitment Therapy) 86t
stress and crisis management 86t
success factors, Doctors for Doctors mentoring program 142–5
Summary of duties and confidentiality agreement (template) 187
summary of duties (mentors) 72, 139t, 187
    template 187
support services for doctors 15–16, 17, 45f
Survey Monkey (website) 126
surveys (program evaluation) 126–7
    worksheets and templates 202–23

T

tables and figures 8, 40, 42, 44, 45, 49, 64, 80, 83, 118, 123, 131, 137, 138, 139–40, 141
teaching hospitals xv, xvi, 24, 37, 173
teamwork in medical practice 7, 13, 19
templates and worksheets 179–205

terms of junior doctor year 44f, 106, 208
3 Cs 60–1, 143
    defined 207
time management skills 5, 13, 18
to-do lists for junior doctors 3
The Townsville Hospital experience 133–72
training 177, 192–7
    mentors (action plan) 138t
Training calendar (template) 192
training delivery and evaluation 88–90
    certificate of participation 196
    sample questionnaires 194, 195
training design (for mentors) 84–8
training 'ready for anything' mentors 83–92, 192–7
    delivery and evaluation 88–90
    follow-up sessions 91, 192
    training design 84–8
training sequences, template for 193
transformational conversations 83f, 85, 86t, 143, 147
    defined 209
transition from medical school to workforce 14, 16, 35, 40, 135, 136
trust, learning activity 89–90

U

understanding mentoring for junior doctors 1–45
unplanned leave management practices 20

V

values 51–2
    defined 209
    examples of 136
vision 42, 50–1, 54, 60, 144
    defined 209
vision formulation, defined 209
Vision, mission and charter worksheet 180

W

ward rounds 3, 5
well-being of junior doctors xv, 7–9, 13, 17, 27, 73, 86t, 121, 123, 135–6, 144, 145
Whyte, Jamie-Lea (mentor), interview 155–6
Wight, Joel (mentor), interview 151–2
work-life balance 9–10, 24
worksheets and templates 179–205

About the Authors

Dianne Salvador and Dr Rachel Collings are the co-founders of Queensland's first hospital-based mentoring program for junior doctors, Doctors for Doctors, established at The Townsville Hospital in 2011.

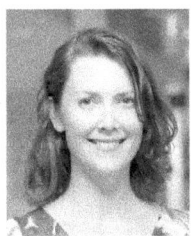

Dianne Salvador

Dianne is a workplace trainer and assessor and a psychologist within medical education. Dianne designs learning experiences for junior doctors, runs medical education events, and teaches design, delivery and evaluation of junior doctor education and well-being initiatives. Dianne graduated from James Cook University in 1998 with a Bachelor of Psychology degree and from Charles Sturt University in 2003 with a Master of Business Administration degree.

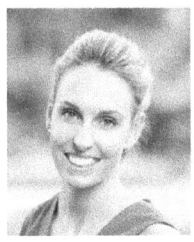

Dr Rachel Collings

Since graduating from James Cook University School of Medicine in 2009, Rachel has had a passion for junior doctor well-being, which she has strongly advocated through her roles on the PMCQ JMO Forum, AMA, The Townsville Hospital Doctors Society, and as a PMCV and PMCQ Accreditation Surveyor. Rachel also has a keen interest in women's health and advocacy and is currently a RANZCOG trainee, specialising in Obstetrics and Gynaecology in Melbourne.

www.ingramcontent.com/pod-product-compliance
Ingram Content Group UK Ltd.
Pitfield, Milton Keynes, MK11 3LW, UK
UKHW051259180426
11947UKWH00020B/1795